Clinical Radiology for Medical Students

Clinical Radiology for Medical Students

K. T. Evans *MB ChB, FRCP, FRCR, FFR RCSI*
Professor of Radiology
University of Wales College of Medicine, Cardiff

I. H. Gravelle *BSc, FRCP, DMRD, FRCR*
Consultant Radiologist
University Hospital of Wales, Cardiff

G. M. Roberts *MD, MRCP, DMRD, FRCR*
Consultant Radiologist
University Hospital of Wales, Cardiff

C. Hayward *MBBCh, FRCR*
Senior Lecturer in Radiology
University of Wales College of Medicine, Cardiff

Butterworths London Boston Durban Singapore Sydney Toronto Wellington

First published, 1982
Second edition, 1987

© Butterworths & Co (Publishers) Ltd, 1987

British Library Cataloguing in Publication Data

Clinical radiology for medical students.–
    2nd ed.
    1. Radiology, Medical
    I. Evans, Kenneth T.
    616.07'57   R895

    ISBN 0-407-01621-X

Library of Congress Cataloging-in-Publication Data

Clinical radiology for medical students.

    Includes index.
    1. Radiography, Medical.   2. Diagnosis, Radioscopic.
I. Evans, Kenneth T.   [DNLM: 1. Radiography.
WN 200 C641]
RC78.C625   1987   616.075'7   87-6373
ISBN 0-407-01621-X

Photoset by Butterworths Litho Preparation Department
Printed and bound in Great Britain by Butler and Tanner, Frome, Somerset

Preface

Diagnostic radiology, including imaging techniques such as ultra-sound and scintiscanning, is an integral component of patient management. It is unfortunate that, partly due to an overcrowded curriculum, students in many medical schools have relatively little instruction in diagnostic techniques and tend to be unaware of the value or limitations of radiological studies.

In this short textbook the radiological appearances in common conditions are dealt with in greater detail. The new imaging modalities have been included in conditions where they play an important role in diagnosis.

The initial chapters are concerned mainly with radiological appearances rather than pathology, whereas the latter part of the text has attempted to define the role of diagnostic radiology in various clinical presentations.

We are particularly grateful to Professor Ralph Marshall and Mr Robert Skinner of the Department of Medical Illustration of the University of Wales College of Medicine and to Dr Robert Davies for enormous help with the illustrations. To our consultant colleagues we owe our thanks for generously giving us material. Finally, we are greatly indebted to Mrs E. Walker for her infinite patience and skill in typing the text.

Contents

Introduction

In order to obtain the maximum amount of information from any radiological investigation it is extremely important that all relevant clinical details concerning the patient's illness be supplied to the radiologist. These should include the present or any former occupation as this may have considerable bearing on the diagnosis, especially in chest disease. The nationality of the patient or travel abroad, especially in the tropics, can also be of importance when considering a possible diagnosis. Previous surgical operations which may modify an investigation or any treatment, such as corticosteroid or immunosuppressive therapy, must also be included in the information supplied.

It is essential that a previous allergic reaction to contrast medium be brought to the attention of the radiologist, although normally he enquires about this directly from the patient before carrying out a contrast study.

As irradiation is potentially harmful, especially to the fetus, abdominal and pelvic radiographs should not be carried out in women of reproductive age if there is a possibility of pregnancy unless there is an over-riding clinical indication. The developing ovum may also be at risk from irradiation; therefore, unnecessary exposure to radiation should be avoided at all times, and there should always be a good clinical indication when requesting any radiological investigation.

Before commencing on a series of investigations it is important to remember that studies using contrast media which are rapidly eliminated, such as excretion urography, should be carried out before barium examinations.

It is always advisable to discuss any complex medical problem with the radiologist to enable planning of the most appropriate procedures and to avoid unnecessary radiation and expense.

Part 1

Chapter 1

The chest

Correct identification of anatomical structures and a knowledge of their normal variants is vital when examining a chest radiograph: misinterpretation of an opacity due to a normal structure may lead to serious errors in diagnosis. A radio-opaque lesion on the skin or in the thoracic cage will produce an opacity superimposed on the lungfields which may be mistaken for an intrapulmonary lesion. Careful clinical examination will avoid such errors of interpretation.

Chest radiographs are normally taken in full inspiration, the erect patient facing the X-ray film with the beam of X-rays passing in a posteroanterior direction. Patients who are so ill that they must be examined on the ward or on stretchers generally have radiographs of the chest taken anteroposteriorly. It is important to realize that such variations in technique can produce distinctive changes on the radiographs as shown in *Figures 1.1a* and *b*.

Table 1.1 Essential differences between posteroanterior and anteroposterior chest radiographs

	PA Chest	AP Chest
Heart	Close to radiograph, little magnification	Magnified image
Scapulae	Normally rotated away from lungs	Superimposed on lung fields
Clavicles	Cross lungfields about 2 in below apex	Frequently projected above apex of lungs

Radiology of the chest in patients with symptoms

In patients with symptoms such as dyspnoea, unexplained weight loss, cough, fever, haemoptysis or pain in the chest, chest radiographs are essential. The examination is also of value in assessing the spread of malignant disease and in the follow-up of such patients.

Note Routine preoperative chest radiography has been demonstrated to be of no benefit and should not be performed in patients without clinical evidence to suggest chest disease.

1

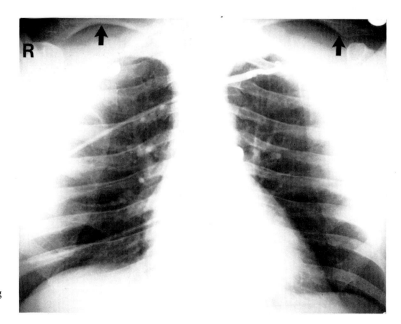

Figure 1.1a AP radiograph showing the clavicles projected above the lung apices, the scapulae overlying the lung fields, horizontal ribs and magnified heart

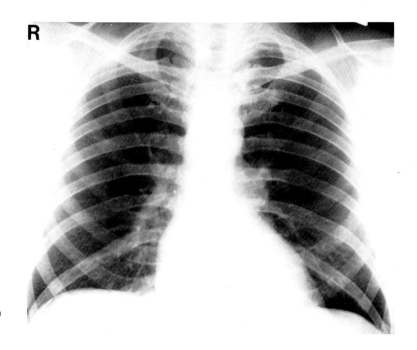

Figure 1.1b Normal PA radiograph of the same patient as in *Figure 1.1a*

Patients with a wide variety of cardiovascular problems require simple as well as complicated radiological studies in order to reach a diagnosis. Radiological investigation is of particular importance if surgical treatment of the disease is contemplated.

Table 1.2 The normal chest radiograph and variations

	Appearances	*Variations*
Diaphragm	Smooth outline, convex upwards	Elevation of left dome due to gaseous distension of stomach
	Sharply defined deep costophrenic angles	Hump on right dome in the elderly (*Figures 1.2a* and *b*)
	Level of sixth rib anteriorly	Fat pad adjacent to cardiac border in obese people
	Right dome about 2 cm higher than the left	
Heart	Assessment of size may be difficult and inaccurate	Geometrical enlargement with AP radiograph, as the heart is further away from the film
	Roughly, the transverse diameter should not exceed half the transverse diameter of the thorax at the level of the diaphragm (or, in an adult, overall diameter should not exceed 15.5 cm)	Apparent enlargement with radiograph taken in expiration
	Two-thirds of the heart lies to the left of the midline	A depressed sternum may displace the heart to the left or compress it, producing apparent enlargement (*Figures 1.3a* and *b*)
Lungfields	Relative transradiancy virtually the same on both sides	Rotation of the patient may produce a marked difference in density between the two sides
	The pulmonary vessels are normally less obvious in the upper zones compared with the lower due to difference in lung volume at these sites. The lower lobe vessels are also larger	Absence of a breast shadow or pectoralis major will produce an increased transradiancy on that side

(a)

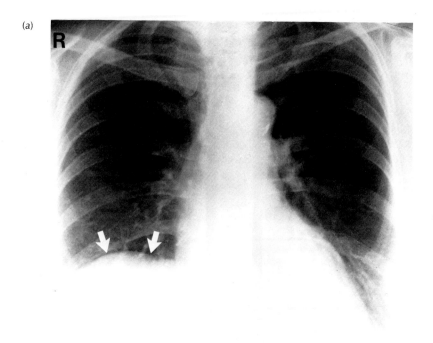

(b)

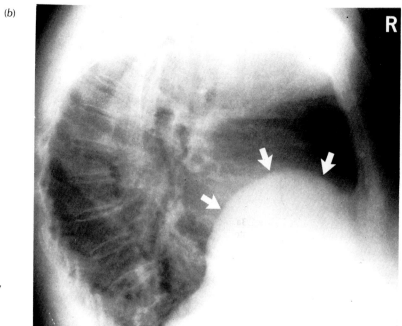

Figure 1.2a and b Anterior 'hump' affecting the right dome of the diaphragm. This is without significance

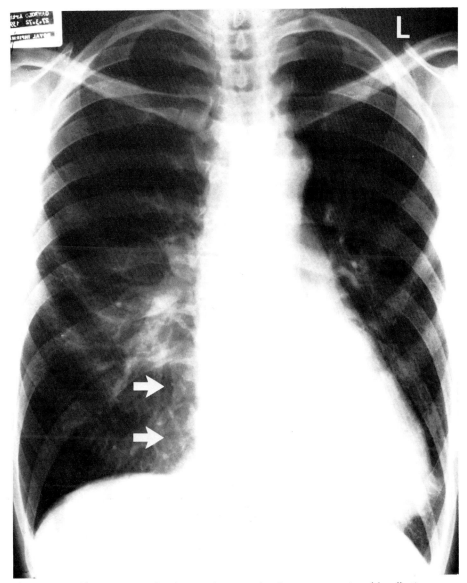

Figure 1.3a and b A patient with a depressed sternum showing gross narrowing of the effective anteroposterior diameter of the chest

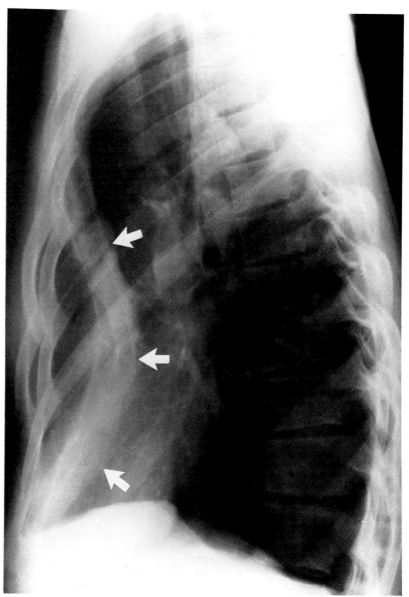

Figure 1.3b

Table 1.2 The normal chest radiograph and variations (continued)

	Appearances	*Variations*
Fissures	Horizontal fissure visible in most adults at the level of the anterior portion of the fourth rib running towards the centre of the right hilum	Accessory fissures – azygos, inferior and, rarely, a horizontal fissure on the left side (*Figure 1.4*)
	Oblique fissures shown in many cases on the lateral film	
Trachea	Lies centrally	May be displaced slightly to the right in elderly patients with aortic unfolding
	Lumen of even width	
Hilar regions	Left hilum lies approx 1 cm higher and is slightly smaller than the right	Left pulmonary artery may be obscured by heart shadow
	Made up of pulmonary artery and central pulmonary veins	
Thoracic cage	Calcification in costal cartilage is common and without significance	Calcification often occurs in irregular fashion and must not be confused with opacities within the lungs
		Cervical ribs and minor congenital rib anomalies are frequently seen
Soft tissue structures	Breast and nipple shadows	Plaits of hair (*Figure 1.5*)
		Clothing
		Artefacts on film
Lateral chest radiograph	The lungs are transradiant behind the sternum and in the lower zones posteriorly	Soft tissues of upper arm may cause shadows
	Radio-opaque areas due to heart shadow and shoulders	

Table 1.3 Projections used in chest radiography

Projection	*Indication*
Erect (PA)	Best projection for patients who are able to stand. Sufficient for most purposes

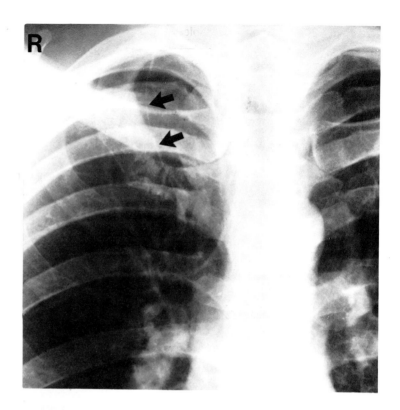

Figure 1.4   Azygos fissure

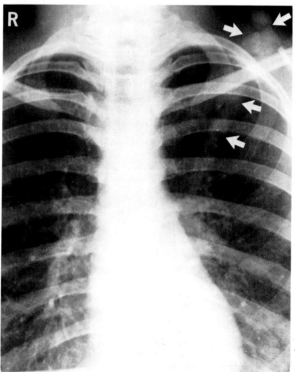

Figure 1.5   Plait of hair overlying left apex. This could be misinterpreted as an abnormality

Table 1.3 Projections used in chest radiography (continued)

Projection	Indication
Lateral	To localize an opacity in the lungs or behind the heart. Not necessary as a routine. Both laterals should never be requested as they are virtually indistinguishable
Erect (AP)	Ward patients
Supine (AP)	Very ill patients or those who are unable to sit up
Tomography	To investigate lesions obscured by overlying structures or to obtain more information about a lesion. Consult with a radiologist before requesting
Penetrated (PA)	Occasionally useful – especially to see cardiac chamber enlargement, e.g. left atrium, and in suspected collapse of the left lower lobe (*Figure 1.6*)
Expiratory	Shallow pneumothorax may become more obvious. Children with suspected inhaled foreign body causing partial bronchial obstruction
Lateral decubitus	To determine whether small collections of pleural fluid are present or in cases of subpulmonary effusions (*Figures 1.7a, b* and *c*)

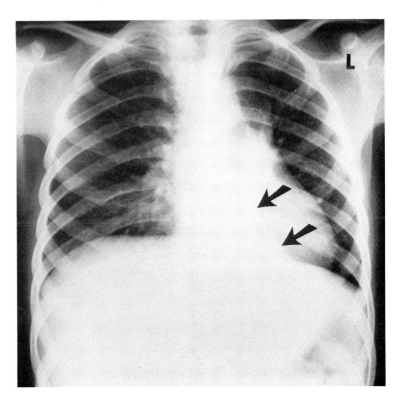

Figure 1.6 Complete collapse of the left lower lobe shown as a triangular opacity behind the heart

(a)

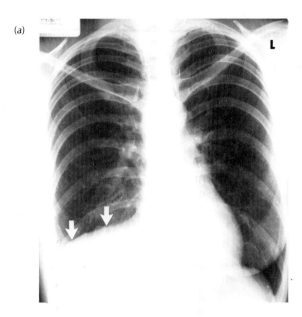

(b)

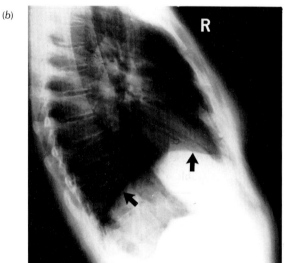

(c)

Figure 1.7a, b and c The posteroanterior and lateral radiographs show
apparent elevation of the right dome of
the diaphragm due to fluid between
the lower lobe and diaphragm
(subpulmonary). The fluid, if free to
move, will lie along the lateral chest
wall on the decubitus film. (c)
Ultrasound confirms the presence of
an effusion (e) above the right dome of
the diaphragm (d)

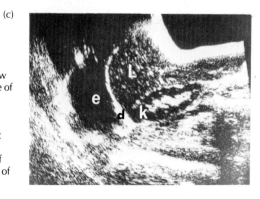

Pulmonary abnormalities

Increased opacification

Radiologically, the normal lung shows branching structures due to the pulmonary vessels. These are clearly seen due to the contrast between the relatively opaque blood vessels and the surrounding air-filled lung, which is transradiant. Air-containing bronchi are not normally seen beyond the main bronchi. However, if the alveoli become filled with fluid, either an exudate or a transudate, the lung becomes opaque to X-rays. In such cases the bronchi, if they remain patent, may be seen as linear transradiancies surrounded by the opaque lung – an appearance known as an air bronchogram. Tumours or inflammatory masses within the lung also produce opaque areas.

If consolidation is present in the right middle lobe or lingula, the adjacent right and left heart borders become indistinct, losing their normally clear outline – this is termed the 'silhouette-sign' (*Figures 1.8a* and *b*). Similarly, the outline of the diaphragm becomes indistinct with consolidation of the anterior basal segments of the lower lobes.

Increased transradiancy

Destruction of lung tissue, as in obstructive airways disease, hyperinflation of lungs in asthma, and a pneumothorax, will produce increased transradiancy.

Table 1.4 Unilateral opacification

	Causes	Radiological features
Pulmonary collapse secondary to bronchial obstruction	Inhalation of a foreign body, especially in children	Displacement of mediastinal structures to side of lesion. Opacification of affected lobes (*Figures 1.9a* and *b*). Elevation of hemidiaphragm. Displacement of hilum or fissures towards collapse
	Carcinoma of bronchus	
	Mucus plug – postoperative	
	Benign tumour, e.g. carcinoid	
Pleural effusion (may be bilateral)	Congestive cardiac failure	A large unilateral pleural effusion displaces the mediastinal structures to the opposite side

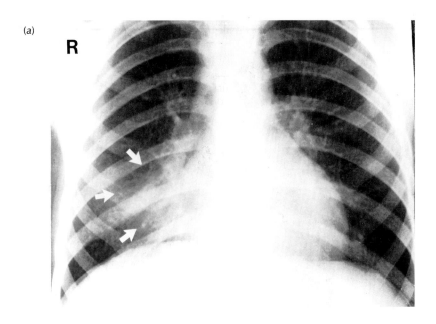

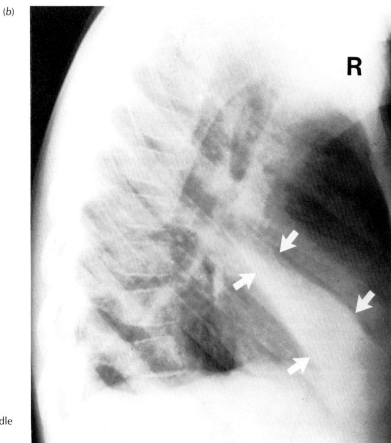

Figure 1.8a and b Consolidation with some collapse of the right middle lobe. Note the right heart border is indistinct

Table 1.4 Unilateral opacification (continued)

	Causes	Radiological features
Pleural effusion (*contd.*)	Malignancy: carcinoma reticulosis	The presence of a large pleural effusion without mediastinal displacement indicates underlying lung collapse. In adults these findings suggest carcinoma of the bronchus
	Hypoproteinaemic states	
	Infection: tuberculous pyogenic	*Figures 1.10a* and *b*
	Following trauma	
	Pulmonary infarction	

Note A fluid level will not be seen unless there is an associated pneumothorax. Occasionally pleural fluid becomes loculated (*Figures 1.11a* and *b*)

Radiologically, a pleural effusion appears to rise along the lateral chest wall. This is more apparent than real. It simply reflects the greater depth of fluid through which the X-ray beam passes, giving increased radio-opacity.

Table 1.5 Large opacities within the lungs

	Causes	Radiological features
Acute	Pulmonary oedema: Left ventricular failure secondary to hypertension, or coronary artery disease	Left ventricular enlargement – usually has characteristic shape – the apex of the heart pointing downwards and outwards
	Mitral or aortic valve disease	Diffuse opacification extending outwards from the hilar regions, which become hazy. (Bat's wing appearance; *Figure 1.12.*) May be unilateral
	Overtransfusion	
		Distension of upper lobe veins
		Septal lines
		Pleural effusion
	Lobar or bronchopneumonia	Opacities of varying size, may be ill-defined, limited to lobar segments or lobules

Note It may be impossible to differentiate radiologically between these acute conditions, and they may coexist, particularly in elderly patients. Clinically unsuspected pulmonary infarcts are extremely common at autopsy.

(a)

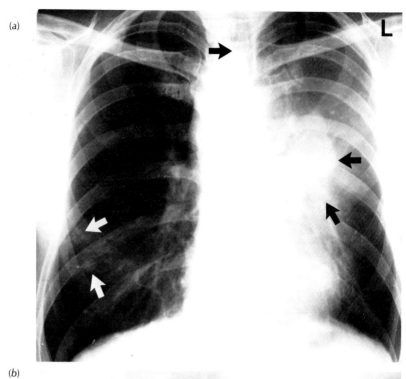

(b)

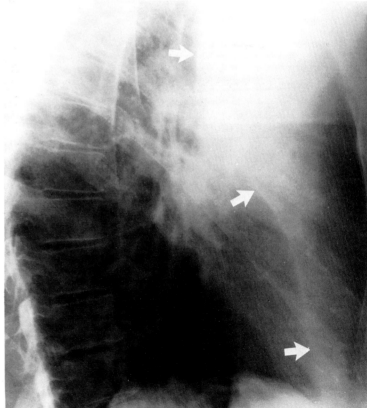

Figure 1.9a and b   Left hilar mass producing collapse of the left upper lobe. The trachea is deviated to the left and the oblique fissure on the lateral view is displaced anteriorly. The left border of the heart is indistinct due to the collapsed lingula. There are metastases in the right lung

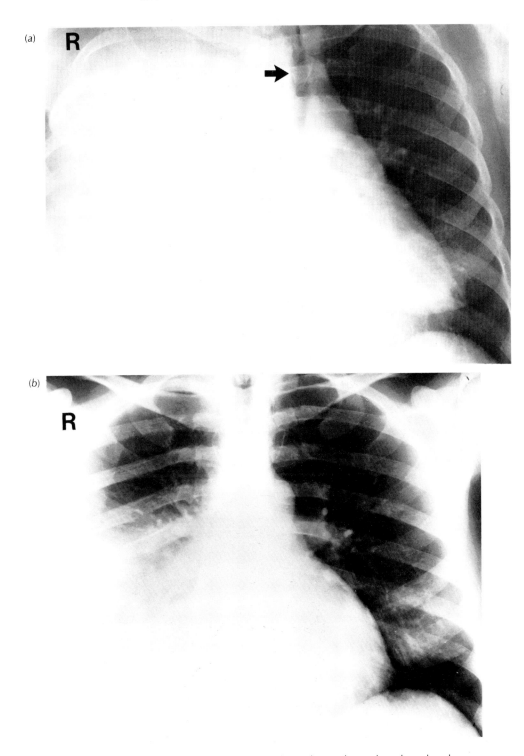

Figure 1.10a and b   Dense opacity in the right hemithorax due to a large tuberculous pleural effusion in a young female patient. The displaced mediastinal structures return to their normal position as the effusion clears with treatment

(a)

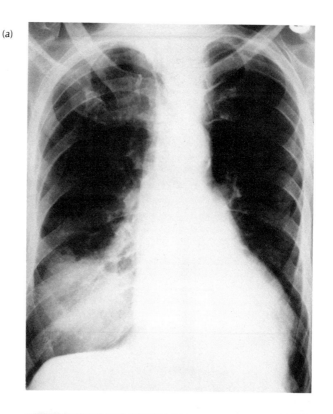

(b)

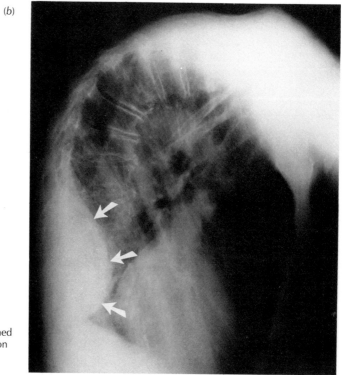

Figure 1.11a and b Dense ill-defined opacity in right hemithorax shown on the lateral radiograph to arise as a result of fluid encysted posteriorly

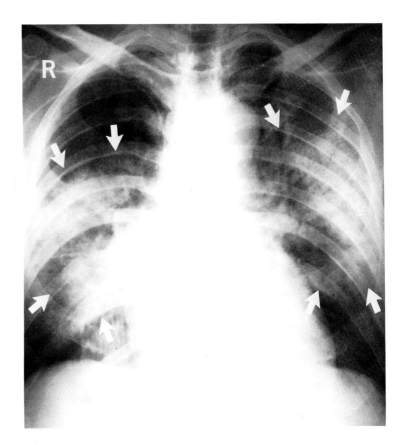

Figure 1.12 Pulmonary oedema. Ill-defined opacification, perihilar distribution. An air bronchogram is visible

Table 1.5 Large opacities within the lungs (continued)

	Causes	*Radiological features*
Acute	Pulmonary infarction	Peripheral opacities, may be linear or wedge shaped, often associated with a small effusion (*Figure 1.13*)
Chronic	Metastases	Generally rounded opacities of varying size (*Figure 1.14*)
	Massive fibrosis secondary to pneumoconiosis	Nodular opacities throughout the lungs, coalescing in the upper lobes. May cavitate (*Figure 1.15*)
	Sarcoidosis	Mediastinal lymph nodes may have regressed

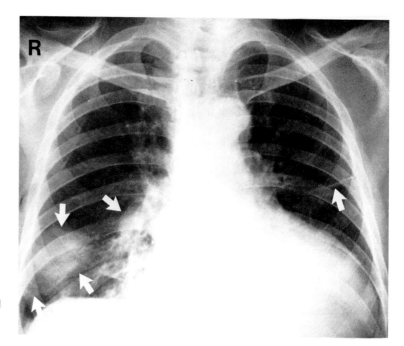

Figure 1.13 Pulmonary infarction. Note wedge shaped opacity at the right base associated with an enlarged pulmonary artery. A linear infarct is seen on the left

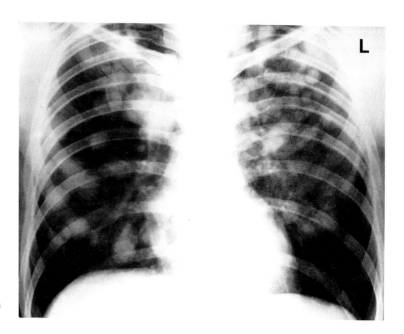

Figure 1.14 Pulmonary metastases showing as multiple well defined rounded opacities of varying size. The primary site in this case was a teratoma of the testis

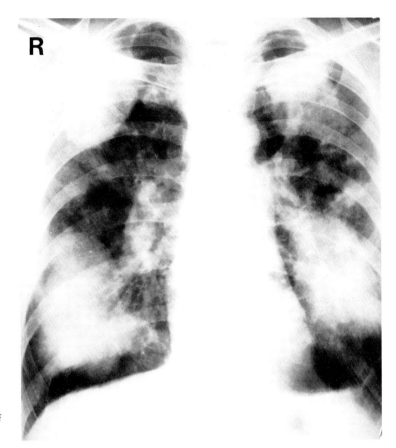

Figure 1.15 Pneumoconiosis with progressive massive fibrosis (PMF). Large, fairly well defined areas of fibrosis in an ex-miner; background of smaller nodular opacities

Table 1.6 Well defined rounded opacities

	Causes	Radiological features
Single	Malignant disease: bronchogenic carcinoma metastasis	Frequently rounded, slightly spiculated outline (*Figures 1.16a* and *b*). May show eccentric cavitation
	Tuberculoma	Frequently contains areas of calcification and satellite shadowing
	Hamartoma	May show characteristic calcification (popcorn)
	Arteriovenous malformation	Large draining veins shown by tomography
	Mycetoma	Fungus ball within existing cavity. Thin 'rim of air' around the lesion (*Figures 1.17a* and *b*)

(a)

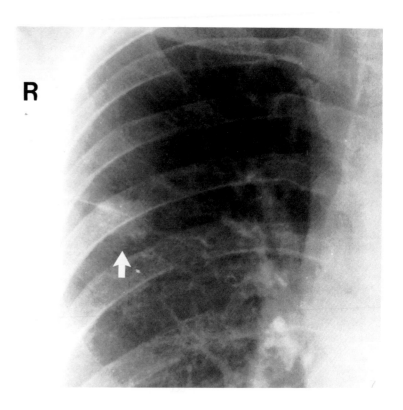

(b)

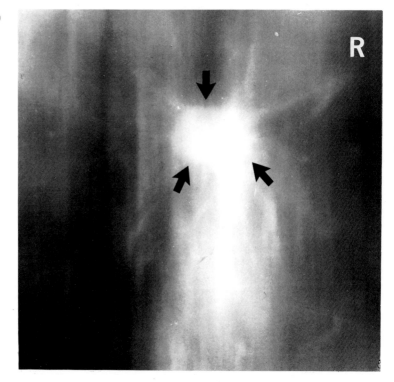

Figure 1.16a and b Bronchial carcinoma. A small solitary rounded opacity in the right mid zone. Tomography of the lesion shows characteristic spiculation

20

Table 1.6 Well defined rounded opacities (continued)

	Causes	Radiological features
Single (*contd.*)	Hydatid cyst	May rupture into bronchus and produce an air fluid level
	Pulmonary haematoma	May cavitate. History of trauma. Associated rib fractures may be present
Multiple	Metastases	Vary in size
	Pneumoconiosis + rheumatoid arthritis (Caplan's syndrome)	Background of nodular shadows. Peripheral rounded opacities of varying size. Sometimes exhibit cavitation
	Sarcoidosis	
	Hydatid disease	

Table 1.7 Multiple small opacities up to 5 mm in size

	Causes	Radiological features
Infections	Bronchopneumonia	Small ill-defined opacities Acute history
	Miliary tuberculosis	Opacities the size of millet seeds
Miscellaneous	Sarcoidosis	May be associated with hilar/mediastinal glandular enlargement. Often history of erythema nodosum (*Figure 1.18*)
	Cystic fibrosis	
	Metastases	
	Haemosiderosis	
Occupational	Pneumoconiosis	Small opacities of varying size. Massive fibrosis in upper lobes depending on severity. Hilar nodes may calcify
	Allergic alveolitis	
	Farmer's lung: acute stage – dyspnoea and wheeze	Small nodular opacities throughout lung fields
	chronic stage— repeated exposure; increasing dyspnoea	Severe pulmonary fibrosis leading to cor pulmonale

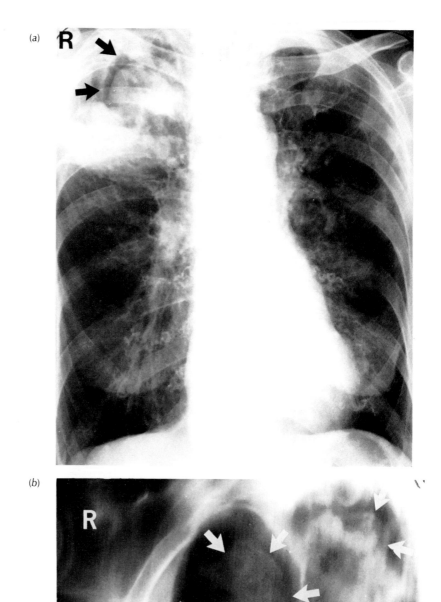

Figure 1.17a and b Mycetomas in the right upper lobe. Both hila are elevated due to long standing pulmonary fibrosis. Tomography shows the rim of air or 'halo sign' around the actual fungus ball within each cavity

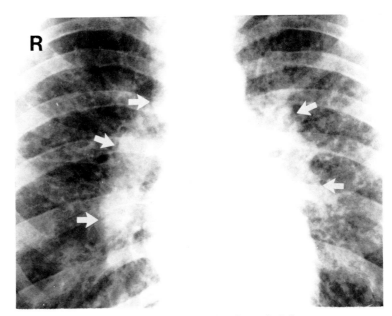

Figure 1.18 Sarcoidosis. Bilateral hilar lymphadenopathy and enlargement of the right paratracheal nodes associated with multiple small nodular pulmonary opacities

Abnormal linear opacities in the lungfields

These must be distinguished from normal vascular shadows. Blood vessels taper towards the periphery of the lung, frequently branch and are tubular in outline.

Table 1.8 Causes of abnormal linear opacities

	Causes	*Radiological features*
Interstitial pulmonary oedema	Left heart failure	Short non-branching septal lines in the periphery of the lungfields (*Figure 1.19*). Septal or Kerley's lines
	Mitral valve disease	
Thickened bronchial wall	Infection, e.g. chronic bronchitis	Tubular shadows. If seen 'end on' appear as small ring shadows
	Oedema	
	Cystic fibrosis	*Figure 1.20*
Fibrous scars	Previous infection	Tend to be thicker and longer than septal lines. Linear scars following infarction are very common
	Pulmonary infarction	
Lymphatic obstruction	Primary or secondary malignant disease	Mass in lung or mediastinum. Linear opacities radiating towards hila and septal lines
	Pneumoconiosis	

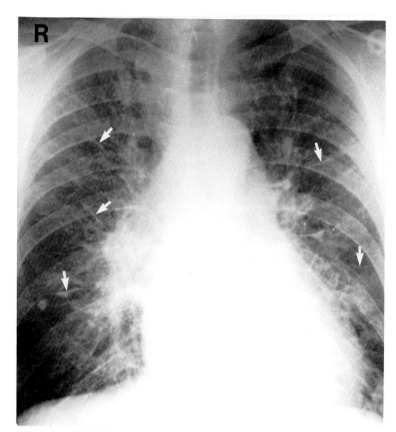

Figure 1.19 Interstitial pulmonary oedema. Patient with left ventricular failure. Note cardiomegaly, numerous septal (Kerley A) lines (arrowed), and ill-defined hila

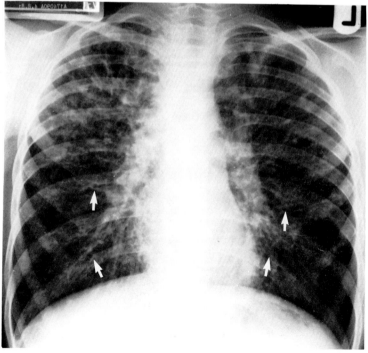

Figure 1.20 Cystic fibrosis showing thickened bronchial walls, extensive inflammatory changes in the lungs and pneumatocoeles

Table 1.9 Localized areas of increased transradiancy within the lungs

	Causes	*Radiological features*
Cavitation	Tuberculosis	Usually in upper lobes. Cavities due to caseation appear within ill-defined opacities. Calcification usually occurs in long standing disease (*Figure 1.21*)
	Bronchogenic carcinoma or metastases, especially squamous cell	Cavity usually small in relation to size of lesion. Often eccentric in position and thick walled (*Figures 1.22a and b*)
	Abscess following pulmonary infection	Cavity within an area of consolidation
Thin walled bullae	Obstructive airways disease	Most often seen at apices
Pneumatocoele	Staphylococcal pneumonia	Frequently multiple, thin walled transradiancies. Disappear as infection resolves. If full of fluid appear as round densities

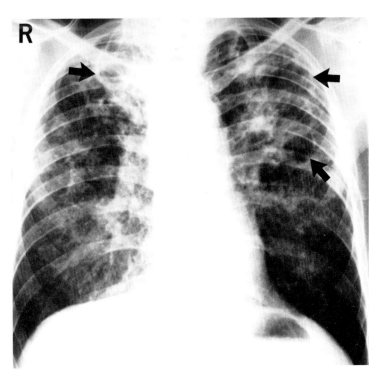

Figure 1.21 Active pulmonary tuberculosis. The disease is mainly in the upper lobes and shows extensive cavitation

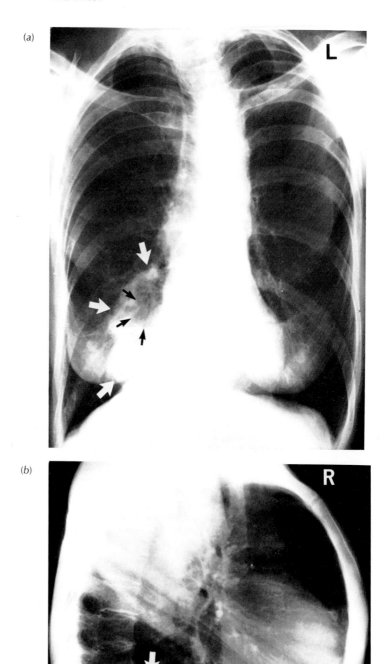

(a)

(b)

Figure 1.22a and b Bronchogenic carcinoma. A thick walled, irregular cavity within the larger mass at the right base

Table 1.9 Localized areas of increased transradiancy within the lungs (continued)

	Causes	Radiological features
Pneumatocoele (*contd.*)	Cystic fibrosis	Come and go with recurrent attacks of infection
Cystic bronchiectasis		Frequently in lower zones. Multiple (*Figure 1.23*)

Table 1.10 Causes of larger areas of transradiancy within the thorax

	Causes	Radiological features
Compensatory over-distension of lung	Collapse of lobe or lung by bronchial obstruction Following lobectomy or pneumonectomy	Increased transradiancy of unaffected lung
Obstructive over-distension	Inhalation of foreign body, e.g. peanut, producing 'ball-valve' effect in bronchus	The lung beyond the obstruction becomes increasingly distended. The diaphragm is depressed, and the mediastinum swings from side to side on respiration
Obstructive airways disease	Chronic air trapping will result in either local or general over-distension of the lungs	Low, flattened diaphragm. Narrow vertical heart. Areas of lung show increased transradiancy with few or absent vessels ± bulla formation. Large pulmonary arteries. On lateral view increased AP diameter of thorax (*Figure 1.24*)
Pneumothorax	Spontaneous, secondary to rupture of subpleural bulla Following chest injury: fractured ribs stab wounds blast injury Postoperative Rupture of subpleural abscess or tuberculous focus	Air within the pleural cavity will produce varying degrees of collapse of the underlying lung. The lung vessels do not pass out to the chest wall (*Figure 1.25*). Occasionally the pneumothorax may be under tension as a result of the 'flap valve' effect. The mediastinal structures are displaced to the opposite side. A tension pneumothorax represents a medical emergency. A fluid level is shown if air and fluid are present in the pleural cavity (*Figure 1.26*)

Note In patients who have had a mastectomy the affected side is more transradiant.

27

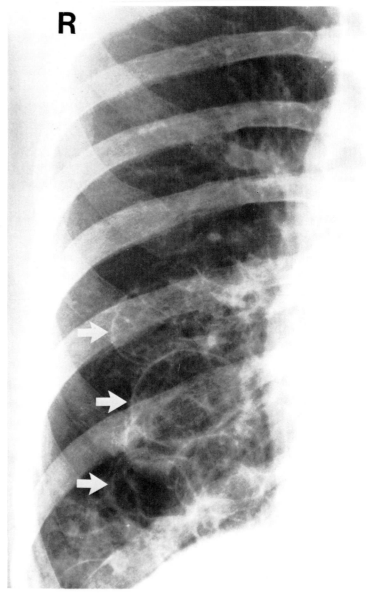

Figure 1.23 Cystic bronchiectasis. Multiple thin walled cysts at the right base – 'soap bubble' appearance. If infected and filled with fluid they appear as dense round opacities

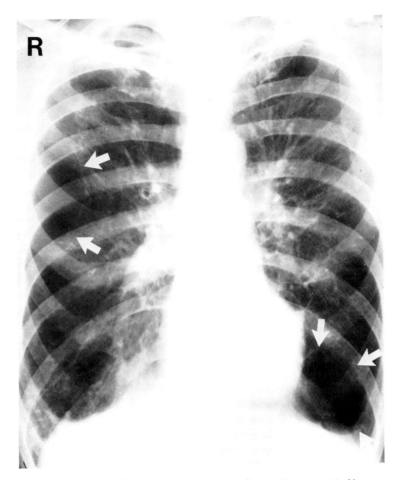

Figure 1.24 (above)   Chronic obstructive airways disease. Narrow, vertical heart, low, flat diaphragm and large pulmonary arteries. Several thin walled bullae are present in the emphysematous lung fields

Figure 1.25 (top right)   Right sided pneumothorax in a patient with neurofibromatosis (n). Transradiant hemithorax, the edge of the collapsed lung is seen adjacent to the right cardiac border, and a pleural fibrous strand is present in the mid zone

Figure 1.26 (bottom right)   Hydropneumothorax. The edge of the partially collapsed lung may be seen and there are no lung markings present in the upper part of the left hemithorax. Because of the air present an air/fluid level indicates the level of the effusion

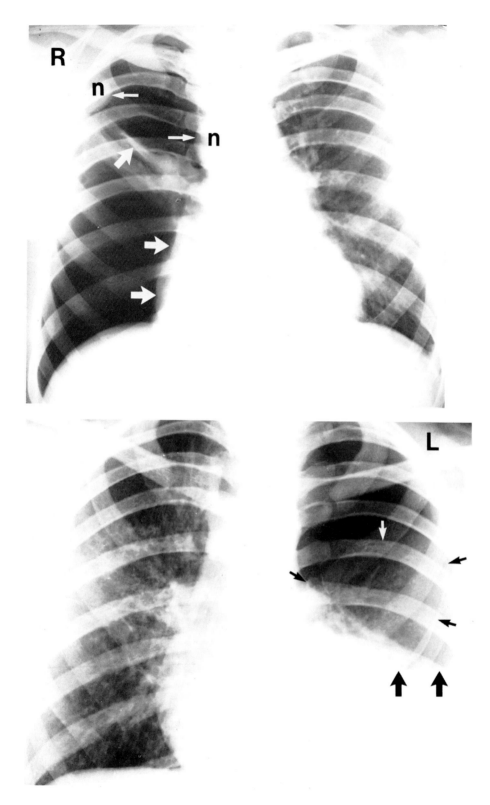

Enlargement of the heart

Cardiac measurement, as stated previously, is imprecise and minor degrees of enlargement cannot be assessed radiologically. For practical purposes, if the maximum transverse diameter of the heart exceeds half the transverse diameter of the thorax at the level of the diaphragm the heart can be assumed to be enlarged. Enlargement of the cardiac chambers, however, can frequently be demonstrated radiologically, and such information can be of great value in diagnosis; e.g. enlargement of the left atrium seen in mitral stenosis.

Mitral valve disease

The classic radiological findings in a patient with mitral valve disease are shown in *Figures 1.27a* and *b*. In uncomplicated mitral stenosis the overall size of the heart is often within normal limits, apart from selective enlargement of the left atrium. Incompetence of the valve will tend to produce considerable enlargement of the left atrium and left ventricle. The haemodynamic changes that occur in the pulmonary vasculature are well illustrated by chest radiology. In severe pulmonary venous hypertension the features listed below may be present singly or in combination.

1. Upper lobe venous distension.
2. Constriction of lower lobe vessels.
3. Septal lines.
4. Pulmonary oedema.
5. Haemosiderosis.
6. Osseous nodules.

Pericardial effusion

A large pericardial effusion will increase the size of the heart shadow, which tends to become globular in outline (*Figure 1.28a*). However, on plain films the appearances are not specific and cannot always be differentiated from cardiac enlargement due to other causes. A pericardial effusion should be suspected if there has been a rapid change in the size and shape of the cardiac shadow in the presence of relatively normal lungfields, provided technical factors have not been altered.

Specific tests used in diagnosis of pericardial effusion include ultrasound and cardiac catheterization (*Figure 1.28b*).

The pulmonary circulation

Increase in the size of the pulmonary vessels, or pleonaemia, occurs in a variety of conditions, especially left to right intracardiac shunts such as atrial and ventricular septal defects (*Figure 1.29*). High cardiac output states, such as thyrotoxicosis and pregnancy, will also cause a generalized increase in size of pulmonary vessels.

(a)

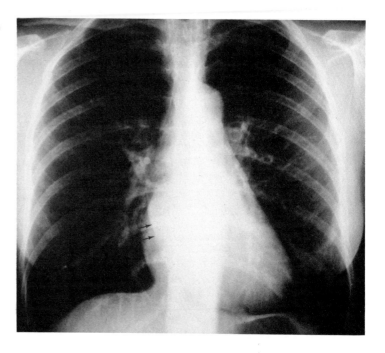

(b)

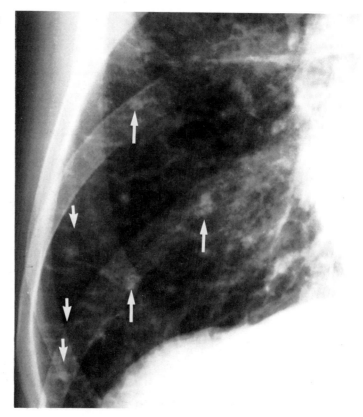

Figure 1.27 Mitral stenosis. (a) Double contour to right heart border due to left atrial enlargement (arrowed). (b) Localized view showing septal lines and osseous nodules present in this patient

(a)

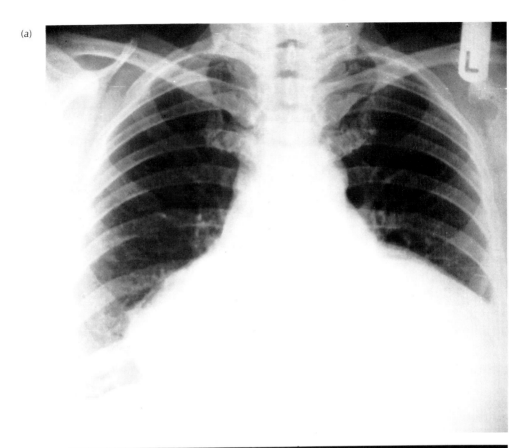

(b)

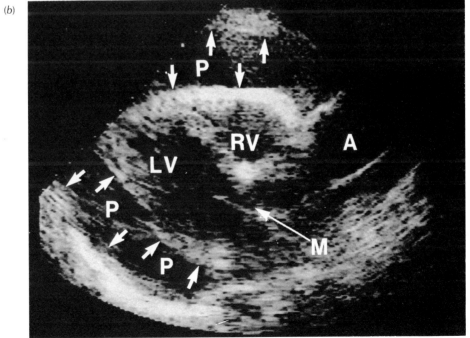

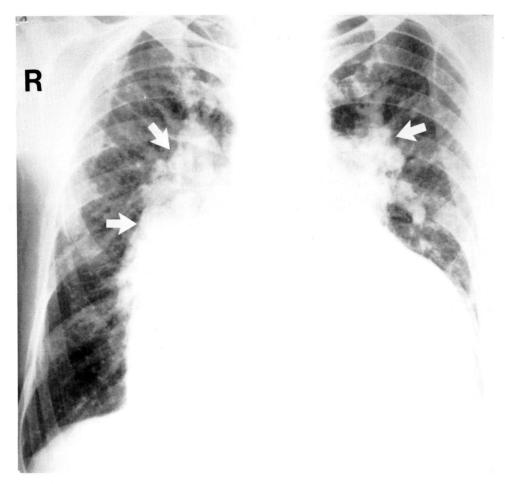

Figure 1.29 Atrial septal defect in an adult – gross cardiomegaly markedly enlarged proximal pulmonary arteries with constriction peripherally indicating reversal of shunt (Eisenmenger's syndrome)

Figure 1.28 (a) (top left) Large cardiac silhouette due to a pericardial effusion. (b) (bottom left) Realtime ultrasound scan through the right ventricle (RV), left ventricle (LV) and aorta (A), demonstrating a large pericardial effusion (P). M = mitral valve

Pulmonary oligaemia may also occur in congenital heart disease, as in cases of right to left shunts, e.g. the tetralogy of Fallot.

Pruning of the peripheral pulmonary vasculature, which produces pulmonary arterial hypertension, may result from thromboembolic disease.

The mediastinum

Note **Radiographs taken with the patient supine show apparent widening of the mediastinum.**

Enlargement of the mediastinal shadow may be due to a variety of causes. Both PA and lateral films are necessary for localization. Tomography, particularly computed tomography, is often helpful in giving additional information.

Having localized the enlargement it is convenient to consider the causes on an anatomical basis.

Table 1.11 Anterior mediastinum

	Causes	Radiological features
Vascular	Unfolded aorta	Very common in older people due to slight elongation of aorta. It is not significant
	Aneurysm secondary to:	
	atheroma	Frequently seen in elderly. Calcification in aortic knuckle
	dissection	Increasing size of aortic outline on serial chest radiographs. May be associated with small left sided pleural effusion
	syphilis	Calcification in the ascending aorta suggests syphilis (*Figures 1.30a* and *b*)
Solid masses	Enlarged lymph nodes	Generally have a lobulated outline (*Figure 1.31*)
	Thymoma	Mass in anterior mediastinum may be associated with myasthenia gravis
	Retrosternal thyroid	Wedge shaped opacity with apex pointing downwards in the superior mediastinum. Trachea or oesophagus may be displaced and compressed (*Figure 1.32*)
Gastrointestinal	Hernia through foramen of Morgagni (rare)	Mass may contain air. Barium studies will confirm

(a)

(b)

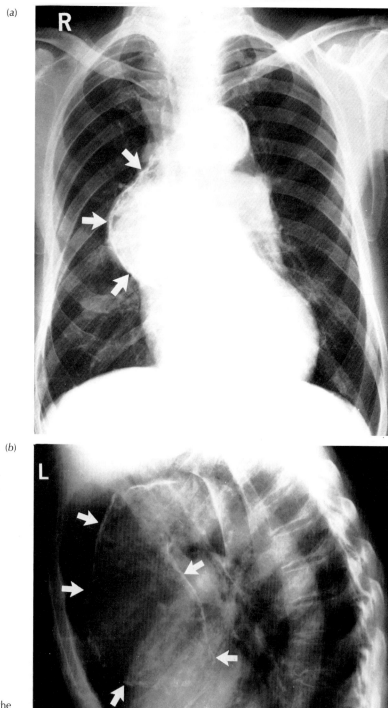

Figure 1.30a and b Aneurysm of the ascending aorta – seen on the PA radiograph as a mass obscuring the right hilum. Calcification in the wall of the aneurysm extending from the valve ring to the arch

Table 1.12 Middle mediastinum

	Causes	Radiological features
Vascular	Aneurysm of aorta	
	Enlarged pulmonary arteries	Project from hila, must differentiate from large lymph nodes. Tomography may be required
Solid masses	Enlarged glands:	Lobulated outline
	reticulosis	May be associated with lymphadenopathy elsewhere
	sarcoidosis	Usually well defined, bilateral and symmetrical
	secondary carcinoma	

Table 1.13 Posterior mediastinum

	Causes	Radiological features
Gastrointestinal	Hiatus hernia	Gas containing structure often superimposed on the heart on the PA radiograph and may contain a fluid level
	Achalasia	Enlargement to the right of the mediastinum from diaphragm upwards, sometimes simulates a large heart. May see an air-fluid level
Spinal	Infection: tuberculous pyogenic	Destruction of vertebral body, narrowing of disc space adjacent. Paravertebral opacity due to abscess. Often multicentric
	Neurofibromata	Stigmata of neurofibromatosis elsewhere. Enlargement of intervertebral foramina – 'dumb bell' tumour
	Neuroenteric cyst	Well defined rounded mass. Frequently associated spinal abnormality

Note The commonest causes of a mediastinal mass are aortic unfolding or aneurysm, hiatus hernia and lymphadenopathy.

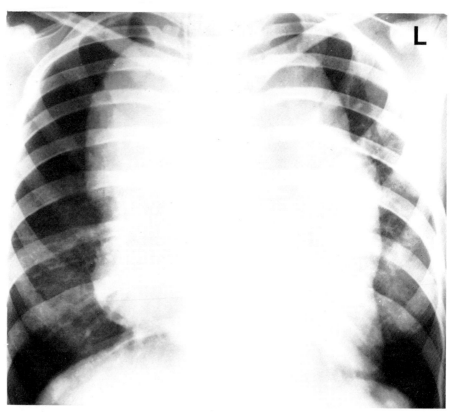

Figure 1.31 Gross enlargement of the mediastinal glands in a patient with lymphosarcoma

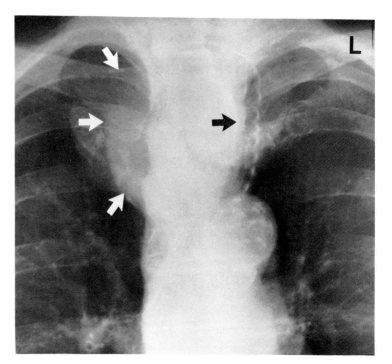

Figure 1.32 Retrosternal thyroid displacing the trachea to the left

Pneumomediastinum

This refers to air in the soft tissue planes of the mediastinum. On a PA radiograph this appears as linear transradiancies which may extend up into the neck, and may also be associated with a pneumothorax or pneumoperitoneum. It occurs occasionally in asthmatics and is an important early sign of perforation of the oesophagus from whatever cause (*Figure 1.33*).

The thoracic cage

Note **Oblique and not lateral radiographs of the chest should be requested when rib abnormalities are suspected.**

Careful inspection of the bony thorax will often provide a clue to disease within the chest and elsewhere. Injury to the chest may result in fractured ribs which may in turn produce a pneumothorax or haemorrhage into the thoracic cavity. Radiologically, this appears similar to an effusion from any other cause. Minor congenital rib anomalies are frequently seen and are of no importance clinically.

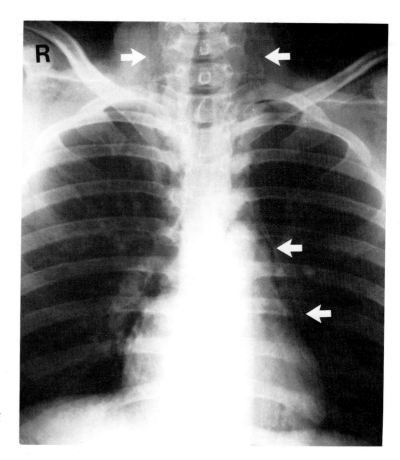

Figure 1.33 Pneumomediastinum. Air is visible in the mediastinum, around the aortic knuckle and can be seen tracking up into the soft tissues of the neck. This patient had spontaneous rupture of the oesophagus

Chapter 2

The abdomen

The normal plain abdominal radiograph

The plain radiograph of the abdomen may present difficulties in interpretation as the contents of the abdominal cavity have similar soft tissue densities and, unlike the structures in the chest, are not sharply outlined by air, with the exception of some parts of the gastrointestinal tract. Use is made instead of the fat layer that surrounds some of the abdominal organs, which, being less dense than the soft tissues, appears as transradiant stripes around such organs as the kidneys. The gas that normally lies within the gastrointestinal tract may give useful information about the presence of disease.

Other structures included on the abdominal film, such as lung bases and the bones, should also be carefully studied. These structures often give important information about the possible cause of the patient's symptoms and may also provide coincidental, but possibly significant, information about other 'non-abdominal' areas and systems.

A chest radiograph should always be obtained in patients presenting with suspected acute abdominal disorders. Some chest conditions, e.g. pneumonia, may mimic an acute abdominal disorder, especially in childhood.

Note Erect abdominal radiographs should not be requested unless an intestinal obstruction or perforation is suspected.

Gas patterns

Normal abdominal radiograph

In the supine abdominal radiograph, gas is normally present in the body of the stomach and in variable amounts in the transverse and other parts of the colon. It is also present in small amounts in the small intestine of adults. Normal gas-fluid levels are usually seen in the gastric fundus on the erect films, occasionally in the first part of the duodenum and in the caecum. In infancy and childhood gaseous distension of the stomach, as well as excessive amounts of intestinal gas, is frequently seen. In supine abdominal radiographs 'pseudotumours' due to fluid in the gastric fundus or duodenal bulb may be present.

41

Abnormal gas patterns in the abdomen

Table 2.1 Absence or diminution of gas

	Causes	Radiological features
Neonates	Oesophageal atresia	Majority of patients with atresias have an associated tracheo-oesophageal fistula below the level of the atresia and, therefore, have normal bowel gas patterns. In those without an associated fistula, no air is seen in the gastrointestinal tract below the level of the atresia. The upper oesophagus may be distended with air. The site of obstruction is shown by taking a radiograph after passing a small radio-opaque tube into the upper oesophagus.
	Diaphragmatic hernia	Usually on the left side. Air containing bowel loops displace the mediastinum and compress normal lung tissue, causing severe respiratory embarassment. Abdomen relatively empty because of large amount of bowel in chest (*Figures 2.1a* and *b*)
	Enterocolitis	Excessive fluid in bowel loops will replace air – may not see air fluid levels on erect radiograph
	Meconium ileus	Speckled gas pattern, this appearance being due to inspissated meconium. Proximally dilated loops of small bowel occasionally with intramural gas

Table 2.2 Excessive gas

	Causes	Radiological features
Infants and children		
Physiological	Air swallowing	
Obstruction	Intussusception	Head of intussusception may be shown as 'soft tissue' mass
Adults		
Mechanical obstruction	Small bowel Postoperative, e.g. adhesions Incarcerated hernia Crohn's disease	Gaseous distension of central loops of small bowel with short fluid levels on the erect abdominal radiograph (*Figures 2.2a* and *b*)

(a)

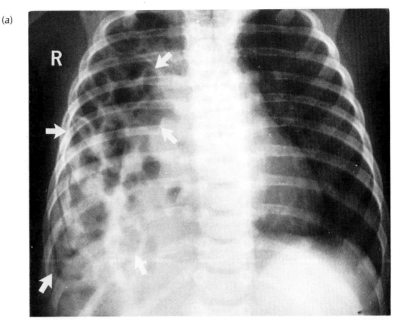

(b)

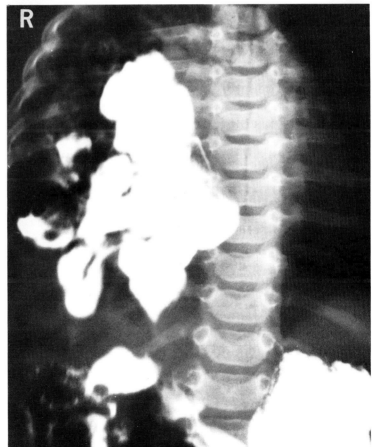

Figure 2.1 (a) Diaphragmatic hernia – 'cyst' like transradiant opacities seen in the right hemithorax. May occasionally be difficult to differentiate from a congenital cystic lung on plain radiographs. (b) Following administration of barium the intrathoracic small bowel loops are easily identified

(a)

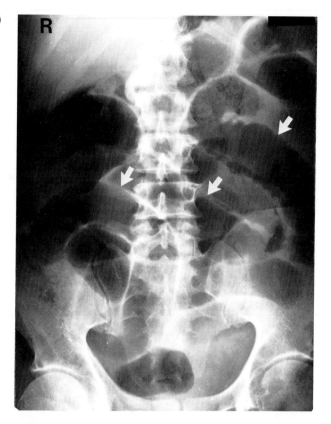

(b)

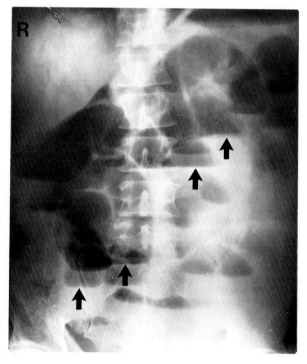

Figure 2.2 (a) Small bowel obstruction. Distended loops of small bowel. Characteristic appearances of jejunum in the left upper quadrant with valvulae conniventes may be differentiated from the more featureless ileum. (b) On the erect radiograph numerous air/fluid levels are seen

Table 2.2 Excessive gas (continued)

	Causes	Radiological features
Mechanical obstruction (*contd.*)	Large bowel	
	Carcinoma – usually left sided	Distension of bowel proximal to obstructing site. Longer fluid levels than those seen in small bowel obstruction
	Diverticular disease, complicated by fibrous stricture formation	
	Volvulus – of sigmoid, caecum	Sigmoid colon – appears as distended loop extending up into the abdomen, resembles an inverted U. Distended caecal pole (generally on a long mesentery) extends towards midline and left upper quadrant
Non-mechanical obstruction	Generalized	
	Following abdominal surgery	Large and small bowel become distended. May be difficult radiologically to differentiate between mechanical obstruction and ileus
	Peritonitis	
	Hypokalaemia	
	Secondary to a mechanical obstruction	
	Localized	
	Acute pancreatitis	Loop of bowel adjacent to area of inflammation becomes dilated – 'sentinel loop'
	Acute appendicitis	
	Pelvic abscess	May see speckled gas shadows due to the abscess
	Vascular occlusion	Area of bowel supplied by occluded vessel is affected

Table 2.3 Abnormal contour of gas containing loops

	Causes	Radiological features
Infants	Pyloric obstruction	Stomach distended with fluid and air. On erect film an air-fluid level is seen in left hypochondrium. Obstruction usually incomplete, so gas is present in bowel

Table 2.3 Abnormal contour of gas containing loops (continued)

	Causes	Radiological features
Infants (contd.)	Duodenal atresia Annular pancreas Bands – congenital	If atresia is complete, no gas present distal to obstruction. Two fluid levels may be seen on the erect radiograph – one in stomach and the other in dilated proximal duodenum, known as the 'double bubble' sign (*Figure 2.3*)
Adults	Crohn's disease	Affects large and small bowel, may see constant narrow segment due to stricture formation, or irregularity of wall suggesting ulceration. Proximal bowel may be dilated, depending on degree of obstruction
	Ulcerative colitis	Narrowed empty colon with loss of haustral pattern. In severe acute attacks 'toxic megacolon' may develop, i.e. colon becomes grossly distended with air. If pseudopolypi are present they appear as soft tissue densities within the colon (*Figure 2.4*)
	Ischaemia	Dilated bowel with fluid levels. Thickened wall due to oedematous mucosa may appear as 'thumb-printing' (*Figures 2.5a* and *b*)

Displacement of gas containing loops

Enlargement of various abdominal organs such as liver or spleen or other abdominal masses may cause displacement of adjacent loops of bowel.

Table 2.4 Extraluminal gas

	Causes	Radiological features
Intraperitoneal	Perforation of a hollow viscus	Appearance depends on amount of free air present; large amount may bulge out flanks. Curvilinear collection of air seen under the diaphragm on the erect chest or abdominal radiograph
	Subphrenic abscess	Air-fluid level under hemidiaphragm, which is elevated. Inflammatory changes at lung base (*Figure 2.6*)

Note Free gas is not invariably present on an abdominal radiograph in a perforation.

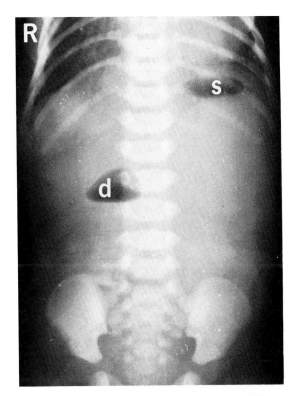

Figure 2.3 'Double-bubble' appearance on the erect radiograph of a neonate with Down's syndrome who has a duodenal atresia – note absence of air in remainder of small and large bowel

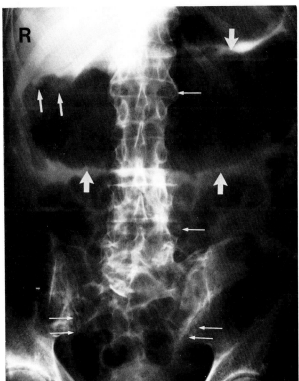

Figure 2.4 Toxic megacolon. Patient with ulcerative colitis. Markedly dilated transverse colon, loss of the normal haustral pattern. 'Pseudopolypi' are seen in the region of the hepatic flexure. Note also associated changes of sacro-iliitis and ankylosis of the spine

(a)

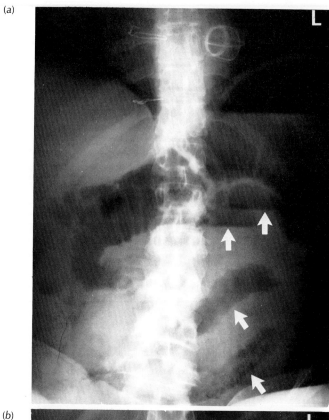

(b)

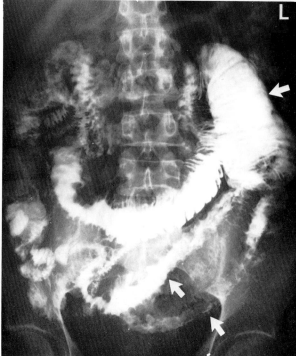

Figure 2.5   (a) Ischaemia of small bowel. Patient with a prosthetic mitral valve who developed occlusion of the superior mesenteric artery due to an embolism. The erect plain abdominal radiograph shows fluid levels in small bowel with abnormal contour of gas containing loops in the left lower quadrant. (b) Barium examination shows the markedly dilated jejunum and evidence of mucosal oedema with 'thumb-printing' in the more distal narrowed small bowel

Table 2.4 Extraluminal gas (continued)

	Causes	*Radiological features*
Bowel wall	Infarction Necrotizing enterocolitis in infancy	Linear transradiancies in bowel wall. May see gas in hepatic portal veins (*Figure 2.7*)
	Pneumatosis coli	Small pockets of gas in wall of colon. May be associated with obstructive airways disease. Patient may be asymptomatic or may present with change in bowel habit or rectal bleeding
Biliary tree	Postsurgical Sphincterotomy Anastomosis between a loop of bowel and the biliary tree	Branching tubular structures in the right upper quadrant. Gas in the biliary tree lies centrally within the liver whereas gas in the portal radicles tends to lie peripherally
	Erosion of gallstone through wall of gall bladder into small bowel	May be associated with gallstone ileus (*Figure 2.8*)
	Perforation of duodenal ulcer into biliary tree	
	Pancreatic neoplasm	May erode into biliary tree
	Infection with gas forming organisms	
Genitourinary tract	Fistula Postsurgical Crohn's disease Trauma	Gas outlines the urinary bladder and occasionally ureters and pelvicalyceal systems
	Infection, e.g. in diabetics	

Abdominal calcification

Many structures in the abdomen calcify, e.g. calcification in the walls of blood vessels and lymph nodes, but these are generally of no significance.

Calcifications seen in other organs such as gall bladder (*Figures 2.9a, b* and *c*) or the renal tract are frequently the cause of symptoms, and also pancreatic calcification (*Figure 2.10*) occurring in cases of chronic pancreatitis.

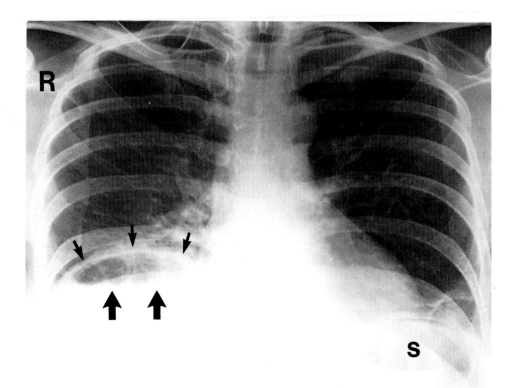

Figure 2.6 Subphrenic abscess. Air-fluid level under the elevated right hemidiaphragm with inflammatory changes at both lung bases

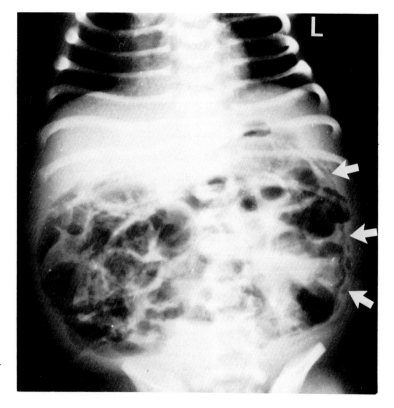

Figure 2.7 Gas in bowel wall of a neonate with necrotizing enterocolitis – both linear and rounded transradiancies are evident, especially on the left side of the abdomen

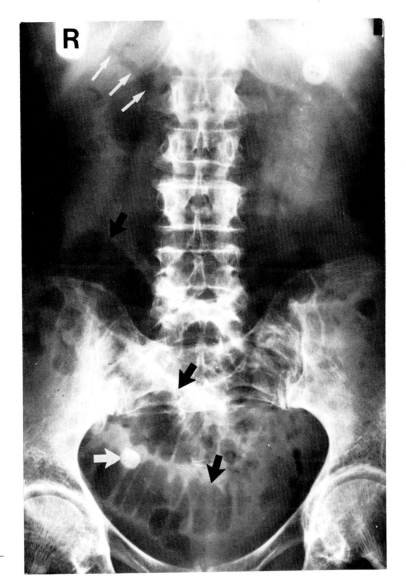

Figure 2.8 Gallstone ileus. Note laminated gallstone in the right iliac fossa and dilated small bowel loops – gas is present in the biliary tree

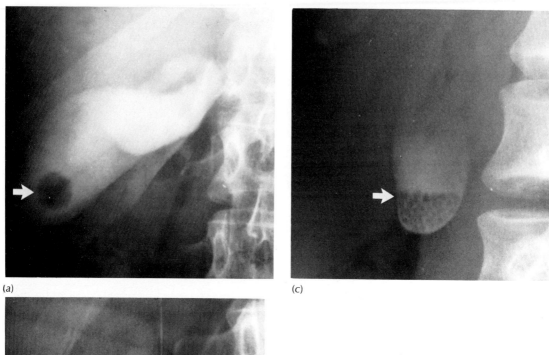

(a)

(c)

Figure 2.9a, b and c Gallstones. Series of oral cholecystograms showing different appearances

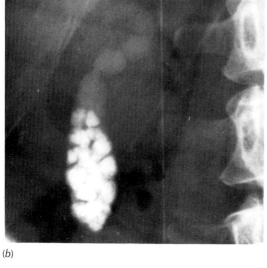

(b)

Figure 2.10 Pancreatic calcification. Punctate calcification extending obliquely across the midline at L.1/L.2 level

Chapter 3

The musculoskeletal system

Radiological findings in bone disease

General points

Note **In these cases listed opposite an isotope bone scan will generally be positive at an earlier stage.**

1. Congenital skeletal anomalies are not uncommon and should not be mistaken for acquired disease.
2. The radiological appearance may be normal even in the presence of established disease:

   e.g. (a) Fracture of scaphoid – sometimes not visible for 10–14 days following injury.
   (b) Osteomyelitis – symptoms precede radiological changes which take time to appear (from 7–14 days).
   (c) Bone metastases may be present and not visible on the radiograph.

3. Bone changes may be non-specific; it may be difficult to differentiate between conditions producing an increase or decrease in bone density.
4. In all cases of skeletal trauma two views at right angles to each other should be obtained as a fracture may only be visible on one of the views (*Figures 3.1a* and *b*).
5. Some diseases affecting bone may cause loss of density, e.g. osteoporosis or bone metastases. Other conditions are characterized by an increase in bone density, e.g. sclerotic metastases from carcinoma of the prostate.

Table 3.1 Conditions characterized by an increase in bone density

	Causes	*Radiological features*
Localized	Bone island – a normal variant	Small area of dense bone, well circumscribed. Most frequently seen in pelvis, upper femora and ribs
	Chronic osteomyelitis	Irregular dense bone, cortical thickening and periosteal new bone formation. May contain sequestra (*Figure 3.2*)

53

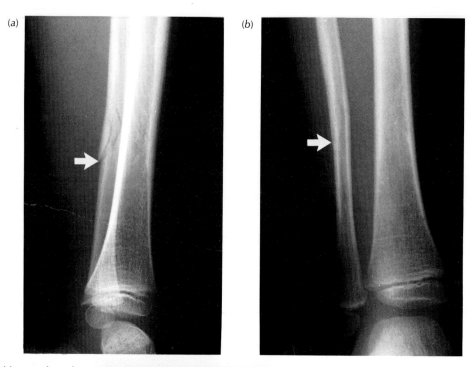

(a) (b)

Figure 3.1 (a) Spiral fracture through shaft of fibula. The fracture line is only visible on the lateral view. (b) The AP view could be considered normal. This illustrates the value of obtaining two views at right angles in cases of skeletal trauma

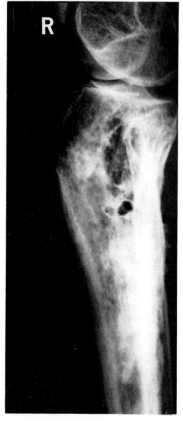

Figure 3.2 Chronic osteomyelitis – upper end of tibia. Abnormal bone texture with areas of increased and decreased density, cortical thickening and irregularity

Table 3.1 Conditions characterized by an increase in bone density (continued)

	Causes	*Radiological features*
Localized (*contd.*)	Others 　Osteoid osteoma 　Pain, chiefly at night, 　usually relieved by 　salicylates	Benign bone tumour. Dense area of bone with central transradiant nidus
	Infarcts	
Localized or generalized	Paget's disease. A common condition	Cortical thickening, coarse trabecular pattern. Long bones become bowed and widened. Pelvis most frequently involved, changes may affect only one half of pelvis. Sarcomatous change may occur in bone affected by Paget's disease (*Figure 3.3*)
	Metastases – osteoblastic 　Prostate – most 　common 　Breast – especially 　following treatment	Ill-defined areas of increased density. May be discrete or produce a diffuse sclerosis (*Figure 3.4*)
	Lymphoma	
	Fibrous dysplasia	
Generalized Congenital	Osteopetrosis	
Acquired	Metastases	May cause a diffuse sclerosis. Frequently a mixed pattern especially in carcinoma of the breast, i.e. mixed lytic and sclerotic appearance
	Myelofibrosis	
	Fluorosis	
	Hypervitaminosis D	

Note In practice metastases from carcinoma of the prostate or breast are by far the commonest causes of bone sclerosis in adults.

Table 3.2 Conditions characterized by loss of bone density

	Causes	*Radiological features*
Osteoporosis:		
Congenital	Osteogenesis Imperfecta (rare)	Marked osteoporosis. Thin cortex, bowing of long bones. Multiple fractures at different stages of healing. Florid callus formation. Fractures may occur in utero (*Figure 3.5*)

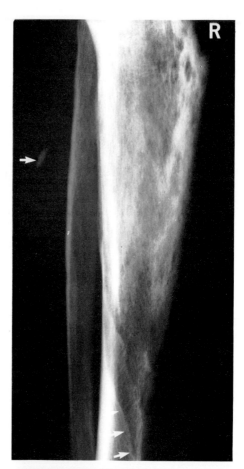

Figure 3.3 Paget's disease affecting upper end of the tibia. Characteristic 'flame' shaped appearance at lower end. Calcification in soft tissues – due to cysticercosis

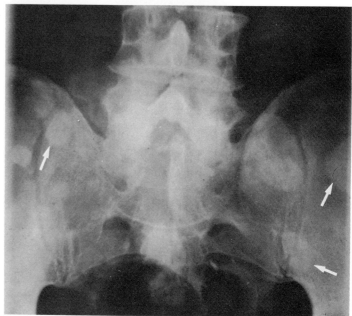

Figure 3.4 Sclerotic metastases in the lumbar spine and pelvis from carcinoma of the prostate

Table 3.2 Conditions characterized by loss of bone density (continued)

	Causes	Radiological features
Acquired Local causes	Disuse Immobilization following a fracture Nerve injury Result of a neuropathy, e.g. poliomyelitis	Affects appendicular skeleton, i.e. the limbs. Patchy loss of density may become uniform, cortex thinned
	Inflammation Infection – pyogenic, tuberculous (*Figure 3.6*)	
	Erosive arthritis, e.g. rheumatoid	Initially peri-articular
	Sudeck's atrophy Post-traumatic Idiopathic	Painful. Intense decalcification of bones, either patchy or even in distribution, affecting distal limbs. Loss of trabeculae, thinning of cortex and soft tissue swelling are all features

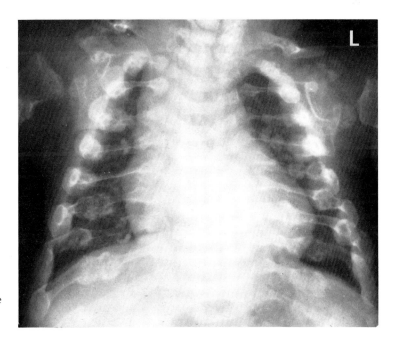

Figure 3.5 Numerous fractures in the thoracic cage of an infant with osteogenesis imperfecta

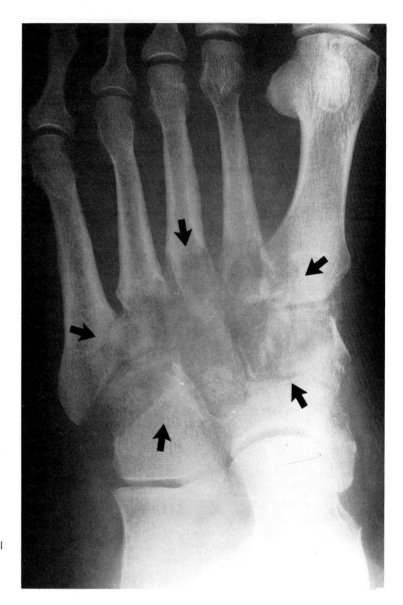

Figure 3.6 Tuberculous infection. Ill-defined area of bone destruction affecting the distal tarsus and proximal metatarsals. No periosteal reaction, which would be evident in pyogenic infection

Table 3.2 Conditions characterized by loss of bone density (continued)

		Causes	Radiological features
	General causes	Elderly, postmenopausal	Loss of density may develop at different rates in different bones. Sharp white 'pencilled' outline to the bones, vertebrae usually maximally affected. Fractures may have wedged appearance and lead to kyphosis. Fractures occur more easily in long bones, especially femoral necks
		Myeloma, leukaemia	
		Cushing's disease, corticosteroid therapy	Fractures seen in ribs, vertebral bodies, pelvis. Tend to be painless. Florid callus formation
		Scurvy – vitamin C deficiency	
	Rickets/Osteomalacia		
		Dietary deficiency – calcium, vitamin D	*Rickets (Figure 3.7).* Infancy and childhood. Characteristic changes confined to growing ends of long bones – wrists, knees, ankles should be examined. Loss of bone density, saucer-shaped splaying of metaphyses, widening of epiphyses. Delay in secondary centres of ossification. Bone deformity. Occasionally periosteal reaction is seen
		Malabsorption states – coeliac disease, postgastrectomy, Crohn's disease	
		Renal Tubular defects – renal tubular acidosis. Glomerular lesions – chronic glomerulonephritis	
		Hepatic – congenital biliary atresia, cirrhosis	*Osteomalacia (Figure 3.8).* Adults. Loss of bone density. Softening of bones leads to deformity and fracture, also biconcavity of vertebral bodies. Looser's zones ('pseudo fractures') may be present and are characteristic. These are transradiant bands of uncalcified osteoid extending from cortical margins across bone, seen especially in ribs, axillary border of scapulae and pubic rami
		Drugs – phenytoin	

Note Assessment of the presence or degree of osteoporosis from a plain radiograph is subjective. Various radiological methods are available to assess bone density more accurately.

Note
1. The skeleton may be apparently normal on a radiograph in the presence of biochemical and histological evidence of osteomalacia.
2. Florid changes are more common in dietary rickets in infants and young children. Changes due to renal disease and malabsorption are similar but often not as pronounced – these are seen more frequently in older children and adolescents.

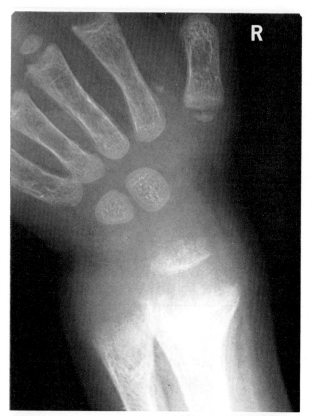

Figure 3.7 Rickets. Right wrist. Cupping and splaying of metaphyses at lower end of radius and ulna. Bones generally demineralized, periosteal reaction present in long bones

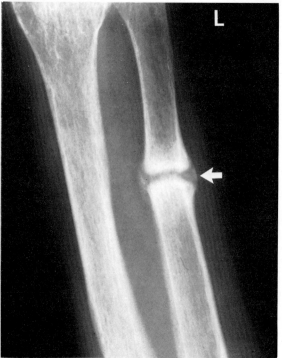

Figure 3.8 Osteomalacia. Characteristic Looser's zone in shaft of ulna

1. Bone changes may occur in all three types. Some changes are more commonly seen in one or other of the three, e.g. 'Brown tumours', rounded transradiant lesions which may expand bone and are trabeculated, are commoner in primary hyperparathyroidism.
2. Presentations of hyperparathyroidism
   (a) Renal tract calcification is the most common radiological feature of hyperparathyroidism. These patients frequently present with ureteric colic as a result of passage of stones, which tend to be radio-opaque due to their calcium content.
   (b) Bone changes occur next in frequency.
   (c) Abdominal symptoms such as dyspepsia and epigastric pain which may or may not be associated with peptic ulceration. Pancreatitis, acute or chronic, is also recognized as being associated with hyperparathyroidism.

Table 3.2 Conditions characterized by loss of bone density (continued)

	Causes	*Radiological features*
Hyperparathyroidism		
Primary	Adenoma, hyperplasia or carcinoma of parathyroid gland	Generalized loss of bone density. Subperiosteal bone resorption seen at radial aspects of phalanges in the hand. Resorption of tufts of terminal phalanges (*Figure 3.9*) Erosion of outer ends of clavicles. Bone deformity and fractures may also occur
Secondary	Chronic hypocalcaemia chronic glomerular disease malabsorption	
Tertiary	Prolonged stimulation of parathyroid glands, which develop autonomous adenomas	

Table 3.3 Transradiant lesions of bone

	Causes	*Radiological features*
Well defined margins	Bone cysts	Usually asymptomatic unless a pathological fracture occurs through them
	Fibrous cortical defect	
	Myelomatosis (see later)	
	Enchondroma	Benign cartilaginous bone tumour. May be single or multiple. Frequently seen in the bones of the hand as expanding, well demarcated lesions with thinning of overlying cortex. May contain calcification. Pathological fractures can occur through them
	Histiocytosis X, e.g. eosinophilic granuloma	Lesions may be single or multiple and not always well defined. Lytic area may involve any bone and periosteal reaction may be present
	Sarcoidosis (*Figure 3.10*)	
Poorly defined margins	Metastases — osteolytic, e.g. breast, kidney, thyroid, lung	Areas of bone destruction which tend to have ill-defined, rather than well-defined, edges. Vary in size and number. Majority occur in axial skeleton. Periosteal reaction is rare

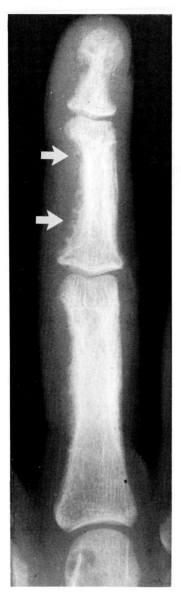

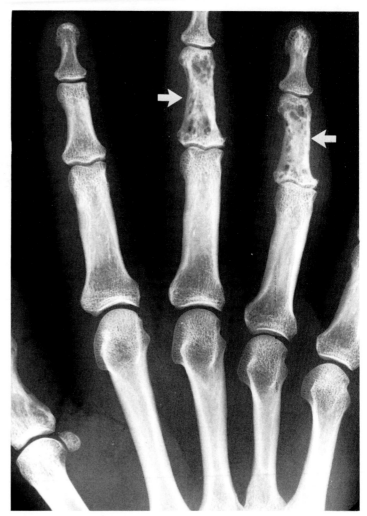

Figure 3.10 Sarcoidosis. Small well defined 'cysts' present in the phalanges. When skeletal changes occur in sarcoidosis they are generally associated with skin lesions

Figure 3.9 Hyperparathyroidism. Subperiosteal bone resorption seen in the phalanges, with resorption of the tuft of the terminal phalanx

Table 3.3 Transradiant lesions of bone (continued)

	Causes	Radiological features
Poorly defined margins (*contd.*)	Malignant primary bone tumours, e.g. osteogenic sarcoma	Affects young people. Most frequently occur around the knee joint, i.e. distal femur and upper tibia. Irregular destruction of bone affecting cortex and extending into the soft tissues, to form a soft tissue mass which may contain new bone formation. Spiculated periosteal reaction (*Figure 3.11*)
	Myeloma	May appear as 'punched out' lesions, frequently difficult to differentiate (radiologically) from metastases. Occasionally solitary, causing bone expansion, i.e. plasmacytoma. An associated soft tissue mass may be present
	Infection	Initially soft tissue swelling with bone appearing normal – later develop destructive changes accompanied by periosteal reaction in pyogenic infections

Note In some cases it is impossible to differentiate infections of bone from neoplastic disease by radiology: this particularly applies if there has been inadequate treatment of osteomyelitis. In such cases it is essential to correlate the clinical, radiological and histological findings.

Periosteal reaction

Elevation and thickening of the periosteum may occur as a response to many of the conditions affecting bone already described, e.g. malignant tumours, infection, trauma, etc. It may also occur physiologically in the neonate.

Hypertrophic pulmonary osteoarthropathy (HPOA: *Figure 3.12*), a condition in which periosteal reaction is associated with finger clubbing, is seen most frequently in patients with carcinoma of the lung, but also occurs with benign pulmonary lesions, e.g. pleural fibroma. The periosteal changes tend to affect the lower shafts of the radius and ulna most commonly, as well as the distal tibia and fibula. These patients may present to the rheumatology department complaining of painful joints.

Skeletal trauma

Radiology is of value to confirm or exclude the presence of a fracture, to demonstrate the type, i.e. simple or comminuted, the relationship of the fracture fragments and to see whether there is any underlying predisposing abnormality of bone.

Greenstick fractures occurring in the growing bones of children heal rapidly, but they may be associated with a more serious epiphyseal injury which can be overlooked. In cases of non-accidental injury in childhood there is frequently evidence of

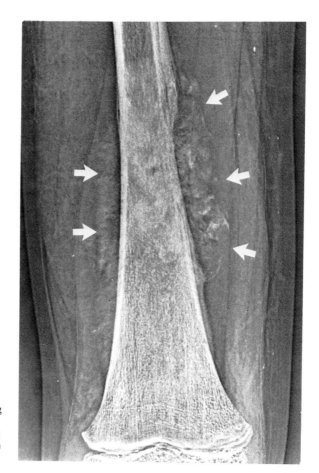

Figure 3.11 Xerogram – right lower femur. Osteogenic sarcoma in a young male. Note unfused epiphysis. Irregular bone texture with a mass extending into the soft tissues. Periosteal reaction on both sides of the femoral shaft

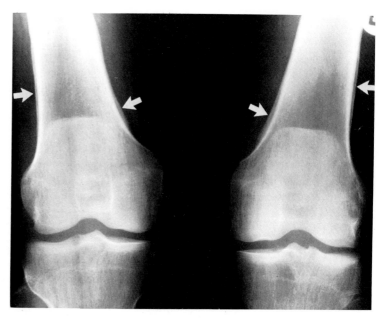

Figure 3.12 Hypertrophic pulmonary osteoarthropathy. Periosteal reaction at the lower ends of both femora in a patient with carcinoma of the lung

multiple fractures at different sites and at various stages of healing (*Figures 3.13a* and *b*).

Transverse fractures rarely occur in normal bone, and if seen, fracture through a pathological area, e.g. a metastatic deposit, should be suspected. 'Stress' or 'fatigue' fractures may occur in normal bone, such as the second metatarsal, as a result of repeated minor trauma, e.g. in athletes, but they are also seen in conditions such as Paget's disease where there is bone softening (*Figure 3.14*).

Difficulties in interpretation of fractures and dislocations

Occasionally, signs of bone injury on a radiograph may be subtle and quite easily overlooked. If these are left untreated there can be serious clinical consequences for the patient, who may be left with severe disability as a result.

Areas in this category include the following:

1. *Fractured neck of femur (impacted)* (*Figure 3.15*). The normal appearance seen in fractures, i.e. obvious discontinuity of bone, is missing. If untreated, avascular necrosis of the femoral head may result.
2. *Posterior dislocation of shoulder and head of femur.* The AP radiograph may appear normal; a second view, e.g. an axial projection, is always required to exclude such an injury.
3. *Translunar dislocation* (*Figures 3.16a* and *b*). The whole wrist except the lunate is dislocated. There are frequently associated fractures present through the radial and ulnar styloid processes.
4. *Monteggia fracture.* The fracture through the ulnar shaft may be seen, but the associated dislocation of the radius at the elbow joint missed.

Skull and vertebral fractures are dealt with elsewhere.

Radiology of joint diseases

On clinical grounds alone it may be difficult to differentiate between the different forms of 'arthritis'. Radiological examination assists and is particularly valuable in assessing the progression or otherwise of the disease.

Osteoarthritis

A degenerative process in which the weight-bearing joints are most commonly affected, i.e. spine, hips, knees. The condition is frequently asymmetrical and may be secondary to previous joint injury or disease. The joints become narrowed due to loss of cartilage, osteophytes are formed at the margins, and there is surrounding sclerosis, frequently with cyst formation. In the hands, the distal interphalangeal and first metacarpophalangeal joints tend to be mainly affected and Heberden's nodes occur, due to osteophytes at the distal interphalangeal joints.

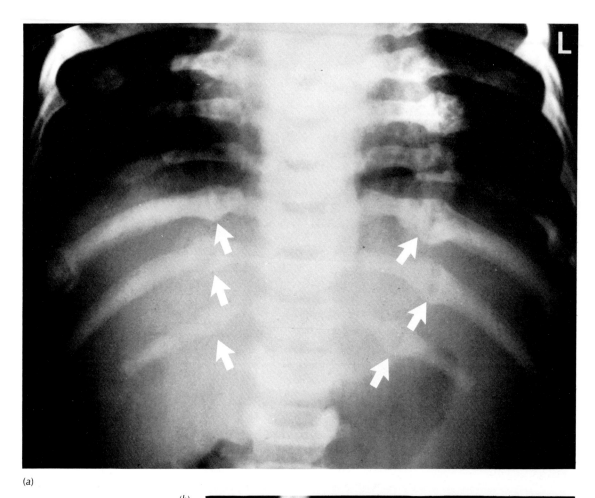

(a)

(b)

Figure 3.13 (a) Non-accidental injury in young child. Numerous fractures at various sites including ribs. (b) Same child also has a fracture through the shaft of radius. Calcified subperiosteal haematoma at the lower end of the humerus associated with injury to the metaphysis in this region

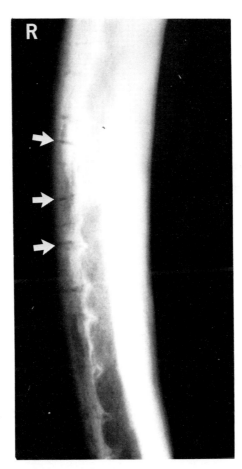

Figure 3.14 'Stress' fractures seen on the convex surface of the bowed femur in a patient with Paget's disease. A pathological transverse fracture may occur through this brittle bone

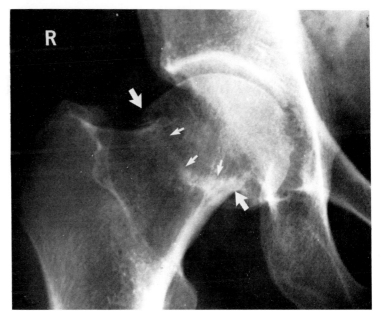

Figure 3.15 Impacted fracture of femoral neck. The dense line (arrowed) indicates the fracture site. This type of fracture is not uncommon in elderly postmenopausal females

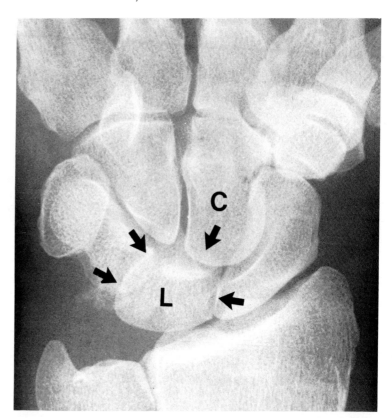

Figure 3.16a Lunate dislocation wrist – AP view – showing the abnormal shape of lunate (L) which appears triangular instead of quadrilateral and loss of 'joint space'

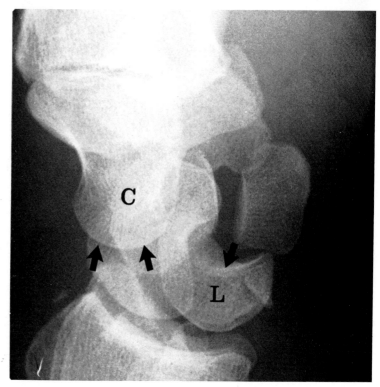

Figure 3.16b The lateral view reveals the extent of injury showing the dislocation of the lunate. Normally the capitate (C) sits in the concavity of the lunate (L)

Rheumatoid arthritis/Still's disease

An erosive arthropathy in which the joint involvement is usually symmetrical. The proximal interphalangeal, metacarpophalangeal and metatarsophalangeal joints and the wrist tend to be most frequently involved. Changes may also occur in any of the larger joints.

Early in the acute phase, soft tissue swelling and periarticular osteoporosis is noted (*Figure 3.17a*). Cortical erosions with narrowing of the joint spaces, eventually leading to subluxation, occurs later (*Figure 3.17b*). If the deformity is very severe the appearance is termed 'arthritis mutilans'. Still's disease is the juvenile form of rheumatoid arthritis, occurring in childhood. Hyperaemia around the joints tends to accelerate epiphyseal maturation and fusion. The cervical spine is not infrequently involved in this form.

Gout (Figure 3.18)

The erosions, which more frequently affect the interphalangeal rather than the metacarpophalangeal or metatarsophalangeal joints, are caused by deposition of sodium biurate crystals and are deeper than those seen in rheumatoid arthritis. Tophi, eccentric soft tissue swellings containing flecks of calcification, are seen around the joints. Osteoporosis occurs much less frequently than in rheumatoid arthritis. Clinically, this condition is more common in males and the patients have elevated serum uric acid levels.

Psoriasis (Figure 3.19)

Resembles rheumatoid arthritis except that the distal interphalangeal joints of hands and feet are affected and there may be resorption of the tufts of the terminal phalanges. These patients tend to have negative rheumatoid factor and there is often associated pitting of the nails.

Haemophilia (Figure 3.20)

An inherited bleeding disorder affecting males in which there is recurrent bleeding into joints. The knees, ankles and ebows are usually involved and the bleeding may be spontaneous or precipitated by minor trauma. These haemarthroses may be large and dense because of the blood content. Eventually there is narrowing of the joint and large bone 'cysts' may develop. Secondary osteoarthritis frequently supervenes at an early age. In some cases ankylosis of the joint occurs.

Neuropathic arthropathy (Figure 3.21)

Impaired pain sensation may be due to conditions such as diabetes, tabes, syringomyelia and leprosy. The associated arthropathy is characterized by marked disorganization of the joint spaces which become subluxed (Charcot's joints).

69

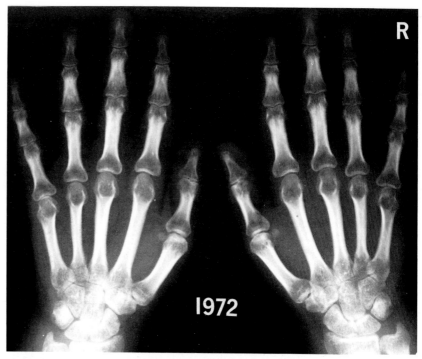

Figure 3.17a Rheumatoid arthritis showing progression of disease. Initially periarticular osteoporosis and soft tissue swelling; no actual erosions seen

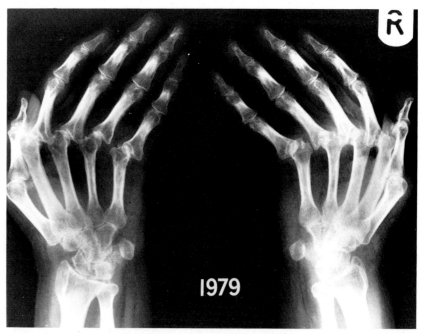

Figure 3.17b Oblique view of same patient. With time, marked erosive changes occur predominantly affecting the metacarpophalangeal regions which are partially subluxed – the phalanges exhibiting ulnar deviation

Figure 3.18 Gout – deep erosions with 'overhanging' edges. Associated with eccentric soft tissue swellings

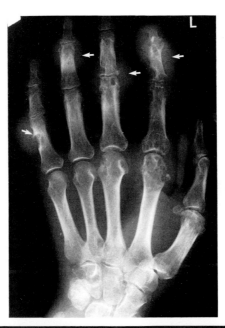

Figure 3.19 Psoriatic arthropathy. Erosions affecting the terminal interphalangeal joints are characteristic of this condition

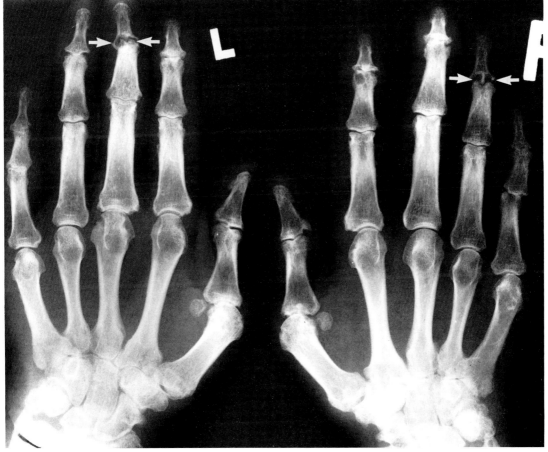

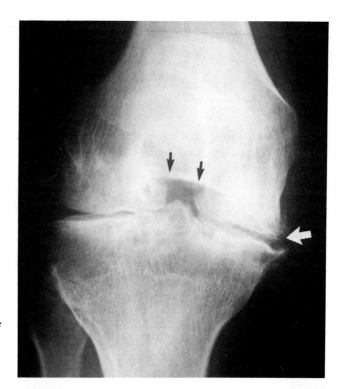

Figure 3.20 Haemophilia. Premature degenerative changes with irregularity of the articular surfaces, squaring of the intercondylar notch and subcortical cyst formation

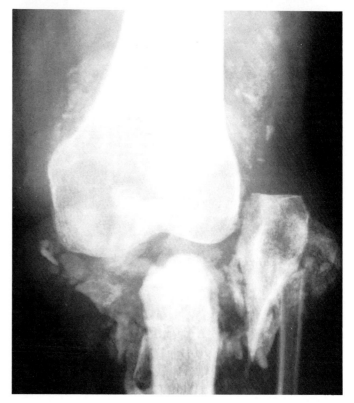

Figure 3.21 Neuropathic joint – left knee. Markedly disorganized with extensive surrounding soft tissue calcification

Avascular necrosis of bone

A condition in which there is fragmentation and sclerosis at the articular surface and bone resorption, leading to loss of normal outline. There are many causes, including trauma which may interfere with normal blood supply, corticosteroid therapy or radiation, deep-sea diving leading to dysbaric osteonecrosis, and sickle cell anaemia.

Perthe's disease affecting the femoral head, which becomes irregular, flattened and dense, occurs mainly in young boys between the age of 5–8 years.

Calcification of intra-articular cartilage and soft tissues

Intra-articular calcification (Figure 3.22)

1. Degenerative, i.e. osteoarthritis – calcification of fibrocartilage.
2. Idiopathic chondrocalcinosis (pseudogout) – affects large joints, calcification of articular and fibrocartilage. Crystals of calcium pyrophosphate found in the synovial fluid.
3. Metabolic – due to conditions such as hyperparathyroidism, haemochromatosis, ochronosis.

Soft tissue calcification

1. Systemic sclerosis (*Figure 3.23*), an autoimmune disorder in which many organs of the body may be affected, including the skin. Calcification is seen in the soft tissues around the tips of the distal phalanges which become absorbed. Muscle calcification also occurs.
2. Parasitic calcification, e.g. cysticercosis – small ovoid opacities lying in muscle with their long axes parallel to the long axis of the limb.
3. Around the hip joints in patients with paraplegia.

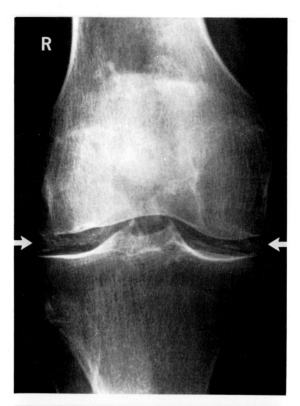

Figure 3.22   Chondrocalcinosis

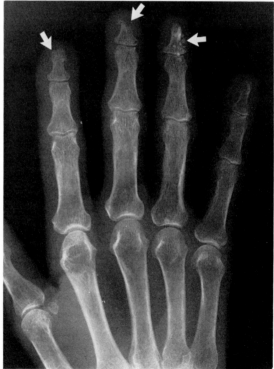

Figure 3.23   Systemic sclerosis. Soft tissue calcification and resorption of tufts of terminal phalanges

Chapter 4   The skull and spine

The skull

Since only the secondary effects of cerebral disease are visible on skull radiographs, e.g. evidence of raised intracranial pressure or cerebral calcification, plain radiography of the skull is frequently unproductive. If the pineal gland is calcified, a space-occupying lesion in one side of the brain may be inferred by displacement of the calcified gland.

The following indications for obtaining skull radiographs tend to be the most productive:

1. Clinical evidence of raised intracranial pressure.
2. Abnormality of size and shape of skull vault.
3. Systemic disorders, such as myeloma, hyperparathyroidism, haemoglobinopathies.
4. Clinical suspicion of pituitary disease.
5. Diseases affecting facial bones, teeth, paranasal sinuses and mastoids.
6. In cases of head injury if a depressed fracture, communication with paranasal sinuses or a foreign body is suspected.

Signs of intracranial disease

Raised intracranial pressure (Figures 4.1a and b)

The radiological signs vary depending on the age of the patient. In children there is often sutural diastasis and increased convolutional markings. The latter is not always of significance.

In adults there may be erosion of the dorsum sellae. This is rarely seen in childhood, but in old age is often seen as a normal variant.

Note
1. Requesting a series of skull radiographs for conditions such as headache, hemiplegia, epilepsy, psychiatric disorders etc. is unlikely to be of value.
2. In middle aged and elderly patients who are being investigated for a possible brain lesion a chest radiograph should always be obtained to exclude a primary lung neoplasm.
3. Anatomical variants in the skull vault such as venous lakes may simulate disease.
4. Normal or physiological intracranial calcification is frequently seen in the pineal gland, choroid plexus and in the falx cerebri.

Table 4.1 Abnormalities of the skull and facial bones

	Causes	Radiological features
Enlargement of skull vault		
Childhood	Hydrocephalus	Sutural diastasis, increased convolutional markings (i.e. 'copper beaten skull')
	Raised intracranial pressure	Bulging of fontanelle in infancy

75

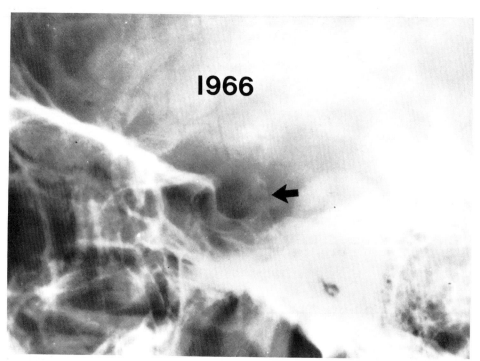

Figure 4.1a   Patient with raised intracranial pressure due to a cerebral tumour. Erosion of the dorsum sellae evident

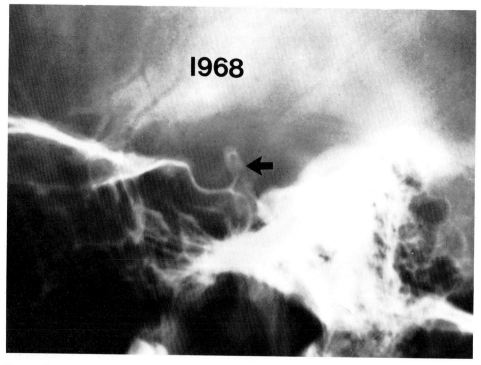

Figure 4.1b   Two years later, following removal of a meningioma, the dorsum sellae has returned to normal

Table 4.1 Abnormalities of the skull and facial bones (continued)

	Causes	*Radiological features*
Adults	Acromegaly	Enlarged frontal sinuses and mandible. Erosion and enlargement of sella turcica
	Paget's disease	Thickened skull vault, increased density of vault and facial bones (*Figure 4.2*)
Increased density		
Localized	Hyperostosis frontalis interna	Frequently seen, especially in females. Symmetrical thickening of bone affecting inner table of vault. Of no clinical significance
	Meningioma	Area of localized sclerosis, may see enlarged vascular groove – due to the feeding artery
	Fibrous dysplasia	Asymmetrical. Affects facial bones, especially the maxilla, and base of the skull
Generalized	Paget's disease	Irregular sclerosis with thickened vault
	Secondary deposits – e.g. prostate, breast	Multiple, ill defined, small dense areas
	Osteopetrosis	Density affects skull vault and base – diffuse skeletal involvement
Lytic lesions		
Childhood	Secondary deposits – neuroblastoma, leukaemia	Variable appearance – sutural deposits may mimic diastasis of sutures (*Figure 4.3*)
	Eosinophilic granuloma (histiocytosis X)	Transradiant defect in vault, frequently edges are 'bevelled'
Adults	Myelomatosis	Rounded transradiancies, tend to be more sharply circumscribed than metastases, but frequently impossible to differentiate (*Figure 4.4*)
	Secondary deposits	Generally multiple ill-defined transradiancies of varying size
	Hyperparathyroidism	Mottled appearance, classically 'pepper pot' skull
	Paget's disease (osteoporosis circumscripta)	Often associated with typical changes of Paget's disease elsewhere in skeleton. Sharply defined transradiant zone, affecting large area of vault

Figure 4.2 Paget's disease. Thickening of skull vault with ill-defined areas of sclerosis affecting both vault and base of skull. The neural foramina may be involved, leading to deafness

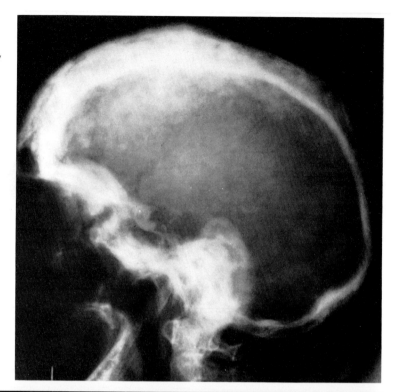

Figure 4.3 Small lytic deposits in the skull vault from a neuroblastoma. Note apparent sutural diastasis due to parasutural deposits

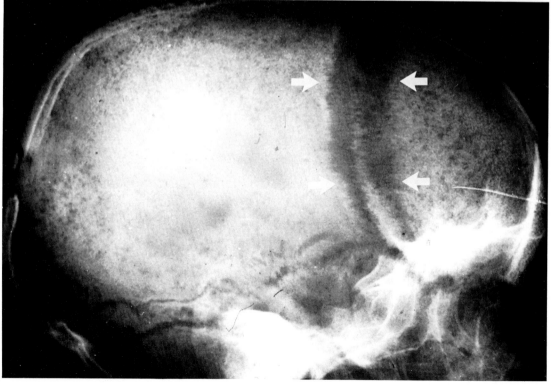

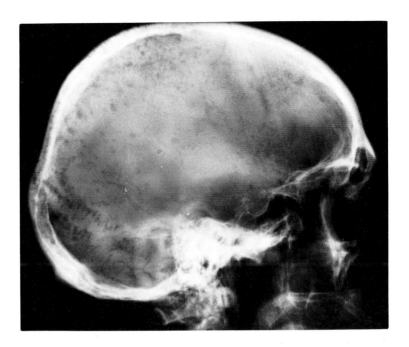

Figure 4.4 Small lytic lesions in the skull vault due to myelomatosis

Table 4.2 Pathological intracranial calcification

	Causes	*Radiological features*
Vascular	Atheroma	Curvilinear calcification, carotid syphon
	Aneurysm	Related to main arteries
	Angioma	Any site, both spotty and curvilinear
	Sturge–Weber syndrome (rare). Clinically, a unilateral cutaneous facial haemangioma is present and epileptiform convulsions occur	Tramline calcification – cortical
Tumours	Meningioma	Calcification in the tumour may be very dense. When related to sphenoid bone or vault may produce localized sclerosis
	Craniopharyngioma	Sella may be deformed. Calcification may be intra- or suprasellar. Such tumours in childhood are more frequently calcified than those occurring in adults

Table 4.2 Pathological intracranial calcification (continued)

	Causes	*Radiological features*
Infection (rare)	Tuberculosis	
	Toxoplasmosis	
	Cytomegalic inclusion disease	
Miscellaneous	Hypoparathyroidism	
	Tuberose sclerosis	

Head injuries

There is generally a poor correlation between the presence of a skull fracture and underlying brain damage. The presence of a fracture very rarely affects patient management unless it is depressed, compound or there is a foreign body present.

Table 4.3 Skull fractures

Types of fracture	*Radiological features*
Linear (*Figure 4.5b*)	Sharp transradiant line, may be straight or angled. May cross a vascular groove, e.g. that of the middle meningeal artery, or affect sinuses, e.g. frontal, and predispose to meningeal infection. Sutural diastasis may occur
Depressed (*Figures 4.5a and b*)	May have curvilinear dense edges. More serious than a simple linear fracture. Tangential views are often necessary for the assessment of this type of fracture
Base of skull	Difficult to detect radiologically. Suggested by the presence of a fluid level in the sphenoidal air sinus, cerebrospinal fluid rhinorrhoea or bleeding from the ear

Note
1. To detect fluid levels in the sinuses in cases of trauma, where the patient is unable to sit up, all lateral skull radiographs should be taken with the patient supine and the X-ray beam horizontal.
2. As brain damage in head injuries is of much greater importance than skull fractures, computed tomography has become of prime importance in order to detect intracranial haematomas.

The spine

Ageing changes commence in the spine relatively early in life. Thus spondylosis, which is a combination of disc degenerative changes and osteoarthrosis of the posterior spinal joints, is very commonly seen in middle aged and elderly subjects.

As intervertebral discs are non-opaque to X-rays, disc herniation cannot be diagnosed on plain radiographs of the spine and myelography will be required (see *Chapter 10*). Only the sequelae

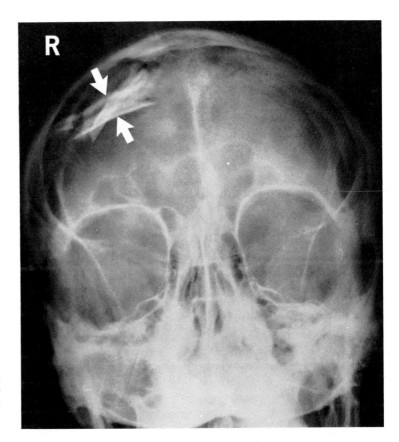

Figure 4.5a Depressed skull fracture – the degree of depression of the bony fragments can be seen in this example on the AP view. Frequently tangential views are necessary

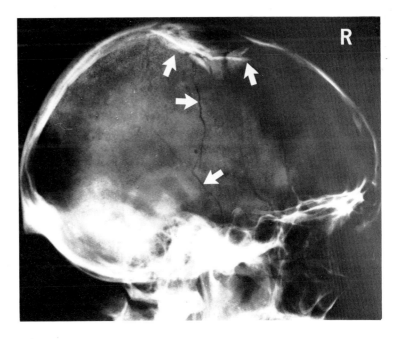

Figure 4.5b On the lateral radiograph a linear fracture is seen running through the temporoparietal region, in addition to the depressed fragment. Compare the fracture line with the adjacent parallel vascular marking

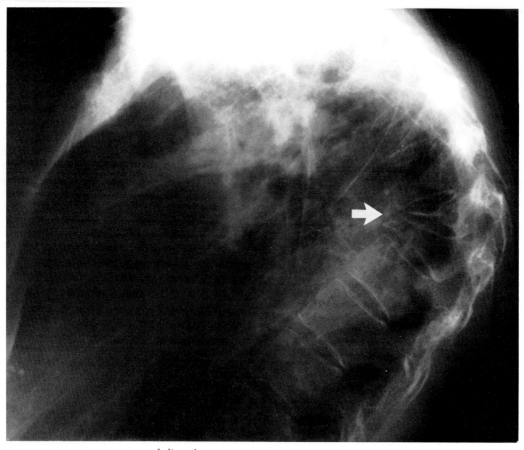

Figure 4.6   Elderly female with osteoporosis. Wedge shaped collapse of mid thoracic vertebrae leading to a marked angular kyphosis

of disc degeneration, consisting of osteophytes, loss of disc height and osteoarthrosis of the joints of the neural arches, are shown on plain films.

Any of the generalized disorders affecting the skeleton, discussed in previous chapters, may also cause changes in the vertebral column, e.g. Paget's disease, metastases (both lytic and sclerotic), myeloma etc. In addition to these pathological processes there are many congenital anatomical variants affecting the spine which generally are of little clinical significance, e.g. spina bifida occulta.

Table 4.4 Abnormal appearances in the spine

	Causes	Radiological features
Trauma		
Minimal	Abnormal bone e.g. osteoporosis, myeloma	Tend to be wedge shaped or compression fractures, involving several vertebrae (*Figure 4.6*) – is of particular importance if associated with dislocation

Note
1. It is important to include all the cervical vertebrae on the lateral view in order not to miss a fracture at C.7 level which may be hidden by the shoulders.
2. Early recognition of a fracture/dislocation is of great importance as the onset of neurological signs and symptoms may be delayed.

Table 4.4 Abnormal appearances in the spine (continued)

	Causes	*Radiological features*
Fracture dislocation	Direct or indirect trauma to normal or abnormal bone	

Loss of density of vertebral bodies

	Causes	*Radiological features*
With disc space involvement	Infection – pyogenic or tuberculous	Transradiant areas due to bone destruction affecting vertebral bodies on either side of the disc space, which becomes narrowed. A paraspinal soft tissue mass due to abscess formation may be present and this often calcifies. With healing, fusion of adjacent vertebral bodies often occurs and some deformity results (*Figures 4.7a* and *b*)
Without disc space involvement	Metastases Myeloma Osteoporosis	Any number of vertebral bodies may be involved. There may be complete or partial collapse – the disc spaces are, however, preserved (*Figure 4.8*)

Sclerosis of a solitary vertebral body

	Causes	*Radiological features*
	Paget's disease	Affected vertebra tends to be larger than the rest – either diffusely sclerotic or may exhibit the 'picture-frame' appearance with sclerosis around the margins. Other bones may also be involved
	Sclerotic metastases, e.g. prostate	May affect only part or whole of vertebra
	Lymphoma	Vertebrae tend to be dense. Large para-aortic lymph nodes may erode the anterior surface of the vertebral body, seen on the lateral view
	Haemangioma	Normal sized vertebra containing dense vertical striations; generally only solitary vertebra affected

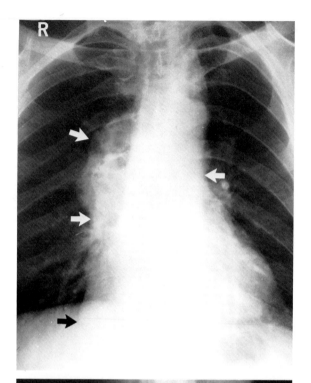

Figure 4.7a PA chest radiograph of a patient presenting with back pain. Note soft tissue mass extending below the diaphragm

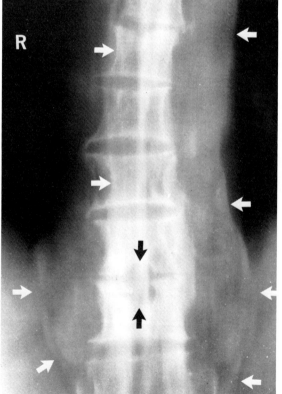

Figure 4.7b Tomographic section of the same patient shows the mass to be paraspinal and associated with a lytic lesion affecting the bodies of T.10/T.11 – there is narrowing of the disc space at this level. These appearances are due to tuberculous infection with an extensive paraspinal abscess, which has caused 'scalloping' of the lateral borders of several thoracic vertebrae

Table 4.4 Abnormal appearances in the spine (continued)

		Causes	*Radiological features*
Neurological disorders			
	Congenital	Spina bifida	Defect in neural arch, widening of interpedicular space. Severe cases associated with a myelomeningocoele
	Acquired	Tumour of the spinal canal Benign, e.g. neurofibroma, meningioma Malignant, e.g. metastatic deposit	Neurological symptoms due to cord compression. Erosion of pedicles due to local expansion of the cord or bone destruction may occur

Miscellaneous causes of back pain

1. Defects in the pars interarticularis (spondylolysis) are not uncommon and these may lead to forward slipping of one vertebral body on another (spondylolisthesis) (*Figure 4.9*).
2. The spine may be affected by many of the erosive arthropathies, e.g. rheumatoid arthritis, Reiter's syndrome, psoriatic arthropathy, etc. The spinal column may eventually become ankylosed.
3. Ligamentous degeneration in conditions such as rheumatoid arthritis may lead to dislocation of one vertebra on another, giving rise to long tract signs (*Figure 4.10*).

Ankylosing spondylitis

A disorder which predominantly affects the sacroiliac joints and spinal column. The sacroiliac joints initially show erosion of the margins and eventually sclerosis and ankylosis. In the spine, the changes usually start in the upper lumbar region. The vertebral bodies become 'squared', the interarticular joints eventually ankylose and characteristic calcification of the lateral and anterior longitudinal ligaments of the spine occurs, i.e. 'bamboo-spine'. The resultant rigidity of the vertebral column makes it liable to fracture with relatively minor trauma. This can have severe neurological consequences especially if the cervical spine is involved.

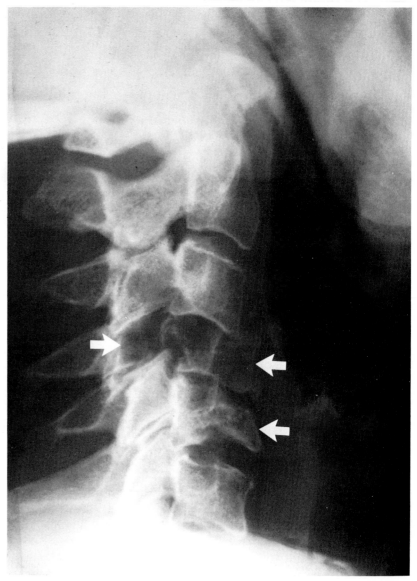

Figure 4.8   Lytic destruction of C.4 and partial collapse of body of C.5 due to metastases from carcinoma of the breast

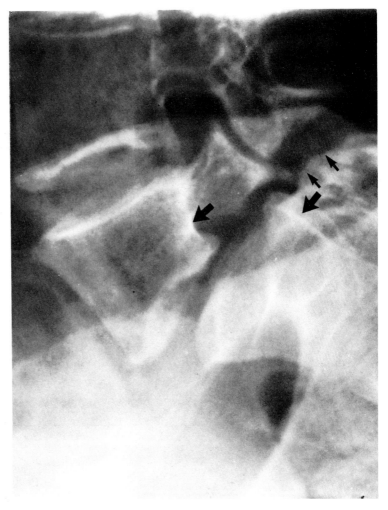

Figure 4.9 Spondylolisthesis – at L.5/S.1. The defect in the pars interarticularis at L.5 and the forward slip of L.5 on S.1 is evident

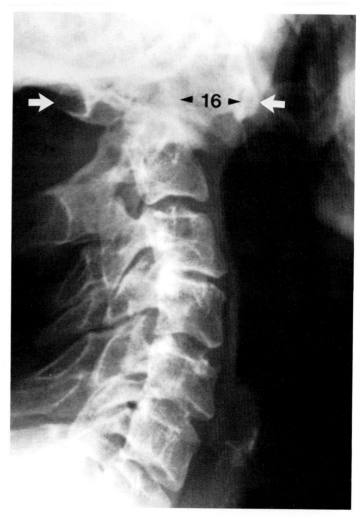

Figure 4.10   Atlantoaxial dislocation in a patient with rheumatoid arthritis.
Note the position of the anterior arch and the spinous process of the first
cervical vertebra in relation to the second. Normally the gap between the
anterior arch and odontoid peg should not exceed 3 mm

Chapter 5

Obstetric radiology
The breast

The size of the pelvis can be determined radiologically (pelvimetry) when clinically there is considered to be cephalopelvic disproportion, or after delivery in cases where a caesarian section has been carried out as an emergency because of disproportion.

Ultrasound in obstetrics

Ultrasound provides an accurate method of diagnosing pregnancy even before the hormone tests are positive and can also be used to estimate the gestational age of the fetus in cases where the patient's dates do not appear to correspond to uterine size. In the very early stages of pregnancy, between 6 and 12 weeks, it is possible to measure the crown–rump length (CRL) of the fetus (*Figure 5.1*) and, after this, the biparietal diameter (BPD) can also be assessed. Both correlate well with the period of gestation and the growth of the fetus throughout pregnancy may be monitored. In this way fetal growth retardation may be detected.

With real time ultrasound scanning, fetal cardiac pulsation is visible from approximately the seventh week of gestation. Fetal limb movement is also seen from an early stage. Twin pregnancy may be diagnosed by ultrasound and many significant fetal abnormalities. These include skeletal abnormalities such as spina bifida, renal abnormalities including cystic disease and various abnormalities of the gastrointestinal tract, e.g. exomphalos.

The localization of the placenta may be determined (*Figure 5.2*), as this is important in cases of antepartum haemorrhage, where there is a suspected placenta praevia, or if an amniocentesis is to be carried out. Unsuspected pathology, such as fibroids or ovarian cysts, may also be discovered.

The breast

Mammography is complementary to clinical examination and enables an earlier diagnosis of breast cancer to be made. It may demonstrate impalpable cancers.

89

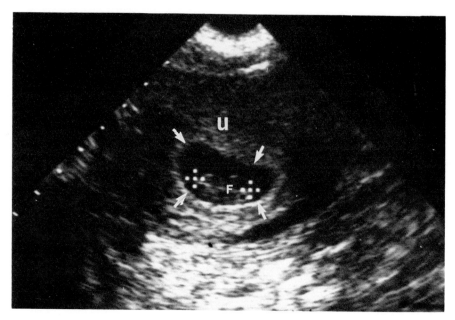

Figure 5.1 Ultrasound scan – longitudinal section; 10-week-old fetus (F) with calipers measuring the crown–rump length. The gestational sac is clearly defined (arrows) within the uterus (U)

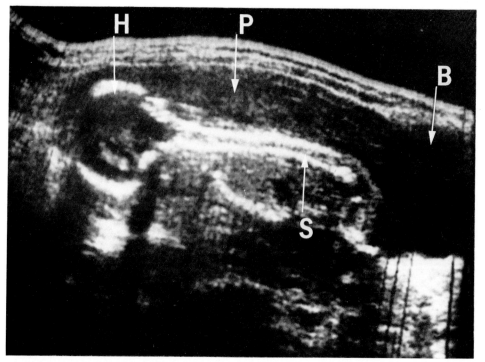

Figure 5.2 Ultrasound scan – longitudinal section; 16-week-old fetus, breech presentation. The placenta (P) is lying anteriorly. The spine (S) is clearly seen as two parallel white lines. The full maternal urinary bladder (B) appears as a 'cystic' structure – without any internal echoes

Mammography may be used to confirm the clinical diagnosis, to clarify clinically uncertain cases and for the preoperative localization of impalpable lesions which require biopsy. It is also useful in periodic assessment of the contralateral breast, following mastectomy and non-surgical therapy for breast cancer.

The main features of breast cancer are the presence of an irregular non-homogeneous, dense mass, sometimes with fine microcalcifications (*Figure 5.3*). The overlying skin may be thickened and nipple retraction seen. Benign lesions, on the other hand, are usually smooth, low density, homogeneous masses and calcification, if present, is coarse (*Figure 5.4*).

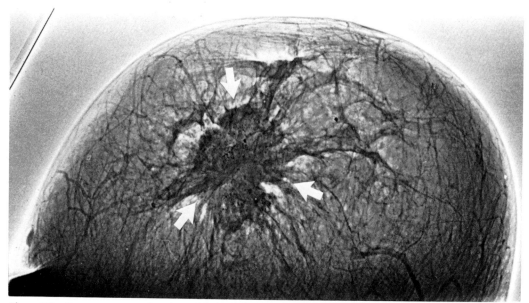

Figure 5.3 Xeromammogram (craniocaudal view). Carcinoma of the right breast. Irregular spiculated mass containing microcalcification

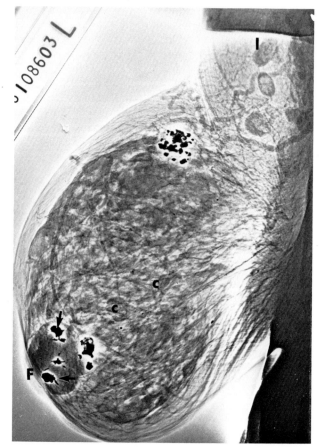

Figure 5.4 Xeromammogram (mediolateral view). Small cysts (c) are present and larger calcified fibroadenomata (F) showing coarse calcification (arrowed), and small discrete lymph nodes (I) in the axilla

Chapter 6   Other imaging procedures

Ultrasound

This is now a well established and widely available imaging technique which has a wide application in clinical medicine. Ultrasound machines are available which can produce both static and dynamic (real time) images. There are many advantages of 'real time' scanning and in the majority of examinations this method is now used. It allows for a more flexible scanning approach and can demonstrate moving structures such as the fetus and vascular pulsation.

One of the major advantages of ultrasound scanning is the differentiation of a solid from a cystic mass. Cystic lesions have the characteristic ultrasound features of low or absent echoes within the cyst and posterior wall echo enhancement (*Figure 6.1*). Solid masses contain echoes throughout (*Figure 6.2*). Areas of calcification, e.g. in biliary calculi, also produce specific ultrasound features with acoustic shadowing distal to the calcification as the ultrasound beam is reflected.

Uses of ultrasound

1. *Pregnancy.* The value of ultrasound in obstetrics has already been discussed (*see* Chapter 5).
2. *Neonate.* Scanning through the anterior fontanelle to visualize the ventricles and surrounding brain if an intracranial haemorrhage or hydrocephalus is suspected clinically (*Figure 6.3*).
3. *Infancy and childhood.* Ultrasound scanning plays an important role in the evaluation of abdominal masses in childhood. It has the advantage of causing no discomfort and requires no special patient preparation.
4. *Adults (Figures 6.4).* Ultrasound is employed mainly in the scanning of intra-abdominal and pelvic contents, but may also be used to examine the eye, thyroid, heart and great vessels and testes. Postoperative subphrenic or other intra-abdominal abscesses may be localized and drained under ultrasound control. Renal and hepatic cysts may also be managed in this way. Fine needle aspiration biopsy of solid masses, e.g. of the

93

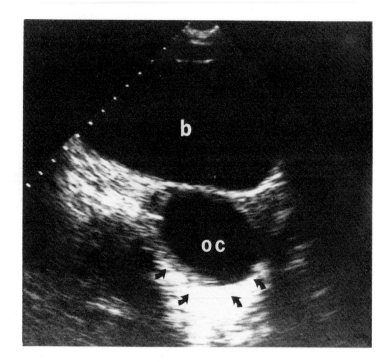

Figure 6.1 Longitudinal scan of the pelvis in an adult female. The anechoic bladder (b) is demonstrated anteriorly with an anechoic simple ovarian cyst (oc) posteriorly. Note the white area indicating echo enhancement posterior to the fluid

(a) *(b)*

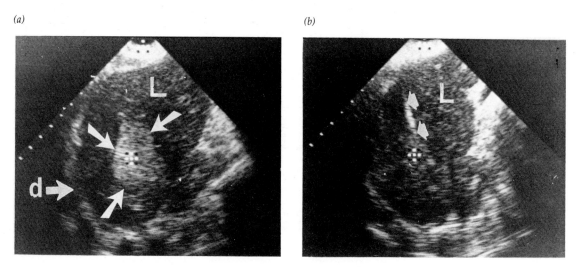

Figure 6.2 Longitudinal ultrasound scans through the liver (L) with the diaphragm posteriorly (d). (a) Echogenic metastases are present. In (b) a biopsy needle (arrowed) has been guided into the centre of one metastatic deposit

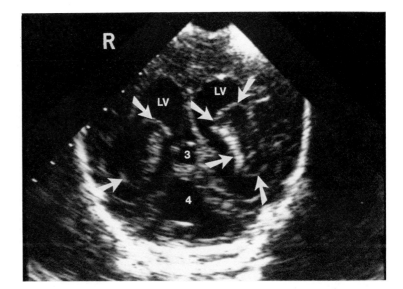

Figure 6.3 Coronal ultrasound scan through the anterior fontanelle of a pre-term infant. There is hydrocephalus with marked dilatation of the lateral (LV) third and fourth ventricles. The hydrocephalus is secondary to intraventricular haemorrhage and the arrows indicate hyperechoic areas due to residual intraventricular haematoma

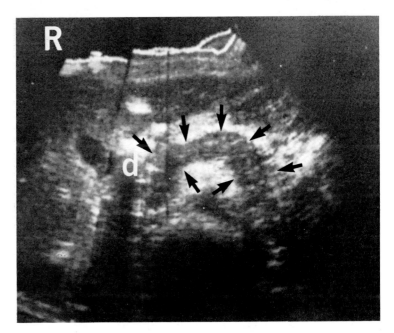

Figure 6.4 Transverse ultrasound scan through the upper abdomen showing a normal pancreas (arrowed) lying anterior to the aorta. The acoustic shadowing to the right is due to gas in the duodenum (d)

liver or pancreas, performed under ultrasound guidance, is an extremely valuable means of obtaining material for cytological study (*Figure 6.2*). This may be used to establish a diagnosis of malignancy and may, in some instances, save a diagnostic laparotomy.

5. *Doppler effect techniques*. A non-invasive method of imaging the vascular system. It allows anatomical and functional information to be obtained from vessels, e.g. detection of stenoses.

Radioisotope imaging

Radionuclide studies are widely employed in all branches of medicine. Both static and dynamic images as well as quantitative information regarding the amount of radioactive uptake in organs may be obtained. Advances in the development of radiopharmaceuticals and recording techniques continue.

Nearly every organ in the body can be investigated by means of radionuclide scanning and adverse reactions to radiopharmaceuticals are rare. The investigations may be performed as an outpatient procedure and radiation exposure is low.

The liver and biliary tree

Abnormalities of size and space-occupying lesions in the liver may de detected following intravenous injection of technetium-labelled colloid particles, which are taken up by the cells of the reticuloendothelial system. Space-occupying lesions, e.g. tumours, do not take up the isotope to the same extent as the surrounding normal liver and are demonstrated as areas with diminished radioactive uptake.

Intravenous injection of a radioisotope (acetanilido-iminodiacetic acid, HIDA) excreted in bile is useful in the evaluation of jaundice, acute cholecystitis and congenital biliary atresia. This is important if acute cholecystitis is suspected clinically, as only radioisotope examination is able to demonstrate the associated blocked cystic duct. Although the demonstration of gallstones by ultrasound or oral cholecystography is possible, this does not confirm the presence of acute cholecystitis.

The renal tract

Radiopharmaceuticals, such as diethyltriamine pentaacetic acid (DTPA) enable quantitative assessment of renal function useful in the investigation of obstructive and reflux uropathy, acute renal failure and renal transplantation. Scanning with a different radioisotope, 2,3-dimercaptosuccinic acid (DMSA), defines the size and position of the kidneys and locates parenchymal defects.

Respiratory system

In the diagnosis of pulmonary embolism, both ventilation and perfusion lung scans are carried out. This involves the inhalation of a radioactive aerosol, such as xenon or krypton, as well as an intravenous injection of technetium-labelled albumin microspheres. In pulmonary embolism, the ventilation scan will be normal but the perfusion scan will demonstrate multiple segmental perfusion defects (*Figure 6.5*).

Skeletal system

Radioisotope imaging with technetium phosphate is particularly useful in the detection of skeletal metastases and acute osteomyelitis which may not be visible on a radiograph. Skeletal metastases may be demonstrated as areas of increased uptake several months before there are radiographic changes (*Figure 6.6*).

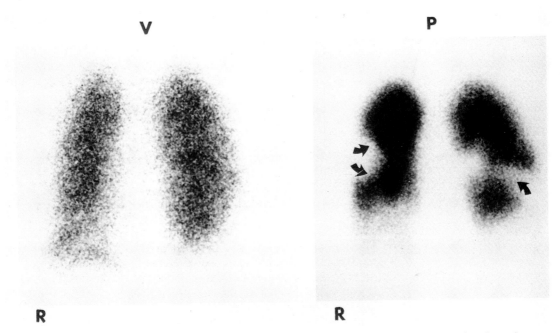

Figure 6.5 Isotope lung scan: the ventilation scan V is normal; P, the perfusion scan of the same patient, demonstrates multiple peripheral defects consistent with pulmonary embolism

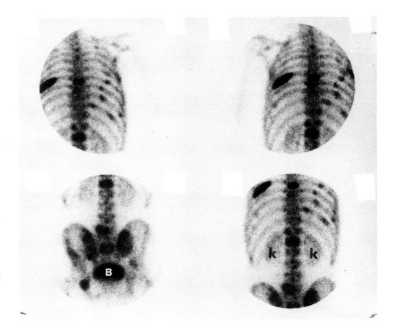

Figure 6.6 Isotope bone scan demonstrating multiple black areas of increased radioactive uptake in secondary deposits from carcinoma of the prostate. It is normal to demonstrate the kidneys k, and the bladder B

Cardiovascular system

Radioisotope scanning provides objective methods for measuring regional myocardial perfusion and detecting myocardial ischaemia.

Computed tomography (CT scanning)

The place of cranial computed tomography will be referred to later (*see* Chapter 10).

Computed tomography allows excellent anatomical detail to be seen in cross-sectional display (*Figure 6.7*). The attenuation values or absorption coefficient of various normal and pathological tissues may be measured. The vascularity of a lesion may be determined by administering an intravenous bolus of water-soluble contrast medium and measuring the degree of 'enhancement'.

'Slices' of varying thickness can be obtained as the X-ray tube rotates about the patient. The photons emerging from the patient are picked up by special detectors.

Thorax

CT scanning has proved particularly valuable in assessment of mediastinal masses and in the detection of small peripheral pulmonary metastases and pleural calcification.

Abdomen

The retroperitoneal area is difficult to image non-invasively except by CT scanning and ultrasound. Computed tomography is especially useful in the detection of lymph node enlargement and adrenal and pancreatic masses, as well as in the investigation of suspected aortic aneurysms. It is particularly useful in detection of intra-abdominal abscesses (*Figures 6.8* and *6.9*). Radiotherapy planning can be carried out with precision and the response to treatment monitored.

Recent developments in imaging techniques

As well as computed tomography, computers are important in nuclear medicine and ultrasound. Computers play a major role in all new imaging techniques including the following.

Digital subtraction angiography (DSA)

The equipment used is a combination of X-ray equipment and high-speed image-processing equipment. High quality images of blood vessels are produced rapidly following intravenous or intra-arterial injection of low volumes of contrast medium. In the correct clinical situation, DSA is easier, faster, safer and less expensive than conventional angiography.

Magnetic resonance imaging (MRI)

The patient is placed in a magnetic field and the response of hydrogen protons in tissues to an applied radiofrequency is measured. Computers process the images in various planes, similar to

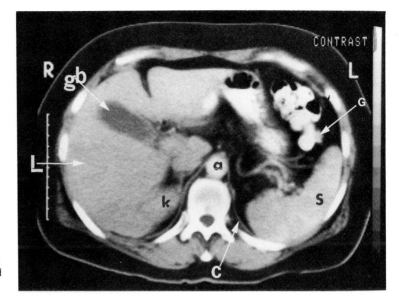

Figure 6.7 CT scan of upper abdomen; normal anatomy. The gallbladder (gb) is lying within the right lobe of the liver L. The crura C of the diaphragm extend down on either side of the aorta, a. The upper pole of the right kidney is visible, k. The splenic vessels are seen extending from the splenic hilum. Water-soluble contrast medium (Gastrografin, G) and gas are present in the colon

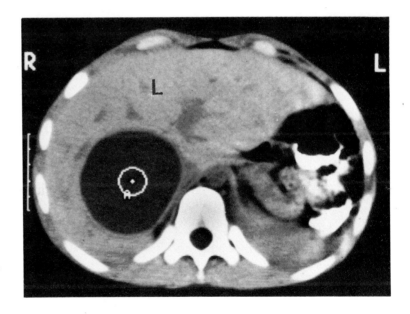

Figure 6.8 CT scan through upper abdomen. Large round mass within the right lobe of liver, L, in a 6-year-old boy. The computer cursor in the centre of mass is measuring the density which is demonstrated to be fluid. This represents a hydatid cyst

those of computed tomography. The brain has been the principal area of clinical interest in MR imaging, although most areas of the body have now been examined. There are a number of advantages of MR imaging of the brain. Unlike computed tomography, bone artefact is not a problem enabling imaging of the posterior fossa. It is possible to easily differentiate between grey and white matter; direct coronal and sagittal imaging is readily achieved and a variety of imaging techniques are available in order to provide anatomical detail or to highlight pathological change (*Figure 6.10*).

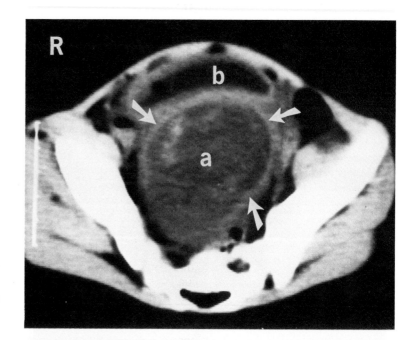

Figure 6.9 Pelvic abscess (a) with a thick surrounding wall lying behind the bladder (b)

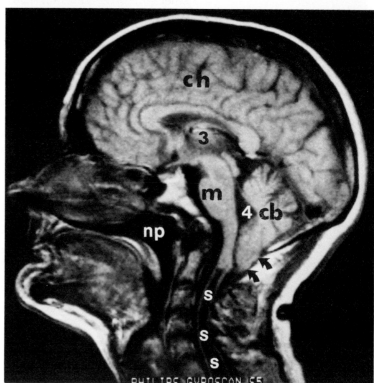

Figure 6.10 Magnetic resonance imaging: midline sagittal scan through an adult brain with cerebellar herniation (arrows) and syringomyelia (S). ch = cerebral hemisphere; cb = cerebellar hemisphere; m = midbrain; 3 = third ventricle; 4 = fourth ventricle; np = nasopharynx

Chapter 7

Part 2

The alimentary tract

Examination of the gastrointestinal tract

Radiological examination of the gastrointestinal tract is of great value in the diagnosis of a variety of lesions. However, a negative examination in the presence of symptoms such as weight loss and anaemia may mean that a lesion has been missed or is too small to be detected. In such cases re-examination after an interval or some other form of investigation is advisable. The complementary nature of radiological and endoscopic examinations is stressed.

Most radiological examinations of the alimentary tract employ a suspension of barium sulphate. Double contrast studies, in which a mixture of barium and air or carbon dioxide is used, can provide fine mucosal detail unobtainable with the single contrast method. The use of image intensifiers and television enables the radiologist to observe peristaltic movements and take radiographs of diseased portions for further study.

In this section diseases of the alimentary tract will be discussed according to their clinical presentation together with their radiological appearances.

Dysphagia

This is a common symptom, but localization of the site of obstruction by the patient is often unreliable. Obstruction at the lower end of the oesophagus may produce symptoms referred to the cervical region. Movement of the column of barium through the upper oesophagus is extremely rapid so a rapid sequence of films or cine radiography is required to enable a detailed study of this region to be made.

Table 7.1 Dysphagia

	Causes	Radiological features
Upper oesophagus	Post cricoid carcinoma	Irregular narrowing, often with a soft tissue mass which may displace the larynx forward (*Figure 7.1*). Inhalation of barium into the trachea frequently occurs during the examination
	Pharyngeal diverticulum	Arise from the posterior aspect of the pharynx. Vary in size, readily demonstrated by a barium swallow
	Oesophageal web. May develop in association with dysphagia and iron deficiency anaemia (sideropenic dysphagia). These webs may also be asymptomatic	Constant filling defect in upper oesophagus (*Figure 7.2*)
	Retropharyngeal abscess	Widening of prevertebral soft tissue space by a soft tissue mass which may contain gas
Mid and lower oesophagus	Carcinoma — Primary	Irregular narrowing of oesophagus
	Carcinoma — Secondary	Invasion from adjacent mediastinal malignancy
	Reflux oesophagitis and stricture formation	Reflux shown on fluoroscopy, frequently associated with a hiatus hernia. Mucosal ulceration may be present; strictures tend to be smooth (*Figure 7.3*)
	Abnormality of oesophageal peristalsis Achalasia	Dilatation of the oesophagus; the lower end is narrowed producing delay in passage of barium into the stomach. Food residue often present in dilated oesophagus at time of barium study
	Systemic sclerosis	Grossly impaired peristalsis, delay in emptying of the oesophagus in the supine position

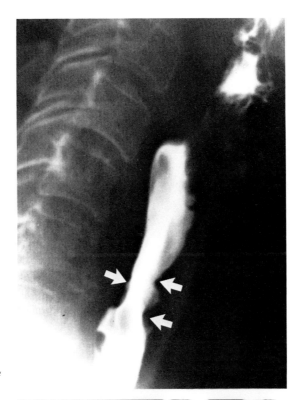

Figure 7.1 Post cricoid carcinoma –
an irregular filling defect encircling the
upper oesophagus

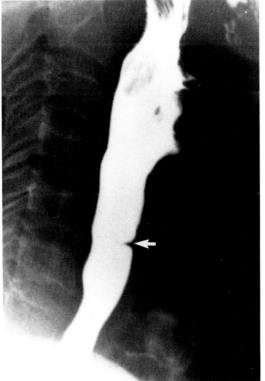

Figure 7.2 Oesophageal web –
appears as a constant sharp indenta-
tion on the anterior aspect of the upper
oesophagus

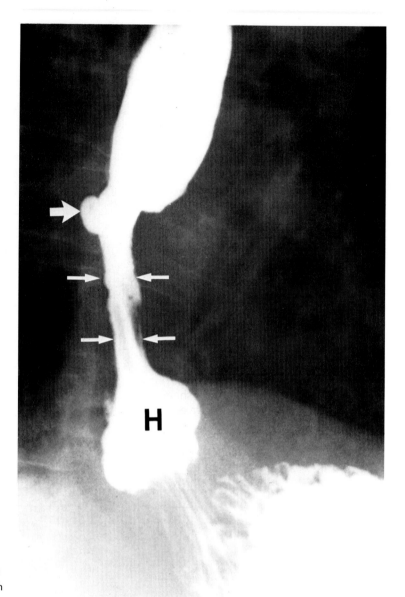

Figure 7.3 Benign peptic stricture of the lower oesophagus in a patient with a hiatus hernia (H). Note also the presence of an ulcer crater (larger arrow)

Table 7.1 Dysphagia (continued)

	Causes	Radiological features
Mid and lower oesophagus (*contd.*)	Stricture following swallowing of corrosive fluids or ingestion of drugs such as emipronium bromide	Severe ulceration may initially be present
	Neurological causes Bulbar palsy Myasthenia gravis	Spill over into the trachea frequently occurs

Haematemesis and melaena

Patients may present following a sudden massive haematemesis with no previous symptoms to suggest disease of the upper alimentary tract. On the other hand, a history of long standing dyspepsia may be elicited. Clinical examination may reveal jaundice, spider naevi or other signs of portal hypertension.

It is now generally agreed that endoscopy rather than radiology should be the primary investigation in patients admitted to hospital with acute bleeding from the upper gastrointestinal tract. Both investigations are often necessary, however, due to their complementary nature.

Table 7.2 Bleeding from the upper gastrointestinal tract

	Causes	Radiological features
Oesophagus	Oesophageal varices secondary to portal hypertension	Worm-like filling defects in lower oesophagus replacing the normal mucosal folds (*Figure 7.4*)
	Mucosal tear in lower oesophagus following forceful vomiting – the Mallory–Weiss syndrome	Non-specific radiology, endoscopy is of value
	Oesophagitis secondary to reflux or corrosives	Irregularity of oesophageal mucosa sometimes associated with an ulcer crater
	Leiomyoma of the oesophagus (rare)	Smooth filling defect. Ulceration may be present
Stomach	Gastric erosions	Small dense flecks of barium surrounded by transradiant halo (*Figure 7.5*)

Note Extensive irregularity of the oesophagus simulating varices may be present in infection by *Candida albicans* (moniliasis), or herpes simplex, especially in debilitated patients and those receiving cytotoxic drugs. Severe dysphagia may be present.

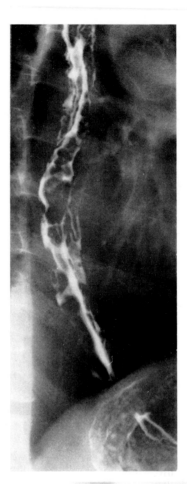

Figure 7.4 Irregular filling defects in the oesophagus due to large oesophageal varices in a patient with portal hypertension

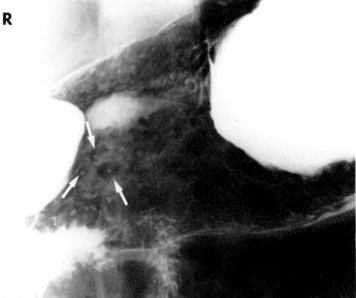

Figure 7.5 Gastric erosions in the antrum appearing as small flecks of barium surrounded by transradiant 'halos'

Table 7.2 Bleeding from the upper gastrointestinal tract (continued)

	Causes	*Radiological features*
Stomach (*contd.*)	Gastric ulcer	(see section on *Dyspepsia*)
	Carcinoma of the stomach	
	Leiomyoma of the stomach	
	Gastric varices	
Duodenum	Duodenal ulceration	
	Invasion of duodenum by pancreatic carcinoma	

Further radiological investigation of patients with bleeding from the upper gastrointestinal tract

1. Investigation where the site of bleeding cannot be determined by endoscopy and barium studies.

    (a) Selective arteriography of the coeliac axis. May show a vascular lesion or demonstrate extravasation of contrast medium into the bowel lumen if the patient is actively bleeding.

2. Investigation of a patient with portal hypertension. Important to determine the patency of the portal vein if 'shunt' procedures are contemplated.

    (a) Arteriography of coeliac axis and superior mesenteric artery. Delayed films will demonstrate the draining veins.

    (b) Splenoportal venogram. Direct injection of contrast medium into the spleen.

3. Occasionally, the isotope technetium sulphur colloid may demonstrate gastric mucosa in a Meckel's diverticulum.

Note Splenoportography is dangerous if there is prolonged bleeding time or ascites.

Dyspepsia

This term relates to symptoms arising from a variety of conditions. Epigastric pain, with or without a relationship to food, is extremely common in association with peptic ulceration, hiatus hernia with reflux, gastric neoplasm, and diseases of the biliary tract and pancreas. It is frequently impossible to arrive at a firm diagnosis on clinical grounds, and radiological investigation, complemented by endoscopy in some cases, is usually necessary.

Table 7.3 Dyspepsia

Symptoms	Causes	Radiological features
Epigastric pain soon after meals	Gastric ulcer ± malignancy	Barium rests in ulcer crater. Often radiation of folds towards ulcer. Sometimes difficult to differentiate benign from malignant ulcers radiologically. Endoscopy and biopsy essential (*Figures 7.6 and 7.7*)
Pain in epigastrium 2–3 hours after meals. Relief with alkali ingestion	Duodenal ulcer	Acute – rest of barium within ulcer crater in first part of duodenum. Occasionally in second part, i.e. post bulbar, narrowing due to spasm. Chronic – 'clover leaf' deformity of first part of duodenum (*Figure 7.8*)
Loss of appetite and weight. Pain may or may not be related to meals and there may be symptoms of anaemia	Gastric carcinoma	Early – mucosal changes in early gastric cancer can be demonstrated by good double contrast barium meals. These cases have been shown to have a good prognosis
		Late – destruction of mucosa. Frequently irregular filling defects within the stomach with advanced lesions (*Figure 7.9*). Diffuse neoplastic infiltration leads to lack of normal peristalsis and distensibility, i.e. 'linitis plastica'
Reflux of acid into mouth. Burning chest discomfort. Flatulence	Hiatus hernia with reflux	On fluoroscopy, reflux of barium into the oesophagus is characteristic. A hiatus hernia often coexists, but is of little significance on its own. Ulceration with or without a stricture may be seen in severe cases

Note

1. **Early gastric cancer can arise within a gastric ulcer which appears benign both radiologically and at endoscopy. Biopsy should be carried out on all gastric ulcers, and repeat examinations are necessary until complete healing has been achieved. Temporary healing of malignant gastric ulcers can occur in patients treated medically.**
2. **Once deformity of the first part of the duodenum has occurred it persists. Radiological re-examination should not be performed unless there has been a change in the patient's symptoms.**

Indications for examination of the small intestine

The small intestine can be examined by giving a barium meal and following the course of the barium through until it reaches the ileo-caeceal valve. Barium may also be introduced via a tube which is positioned at the duodeno-jejunal flexure. The latter is generally regarded as the method of choice, as the examination is wholly under the control of the radiologist and is independent of gastric emptying.

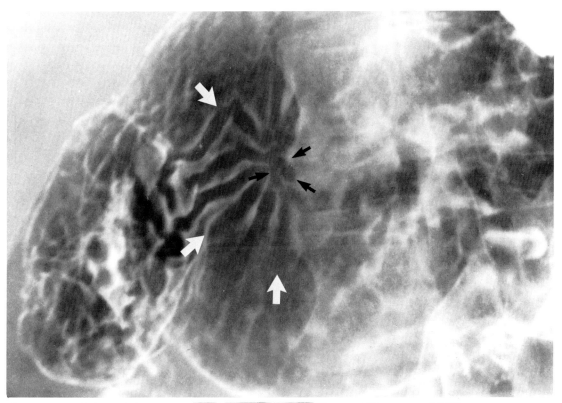

Figure 7.6 Healed gastric ulcer (black arrows) with radiating mucosal folds (white arrows) which extend up to the ulcer crater, suggesting that the lesion is benign

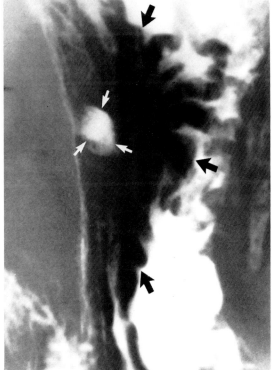

Figure 7.7 Gastric ulcer crater filled with barium. There is amputation of the mucosal folds which may indicate that the ulcer is malignant

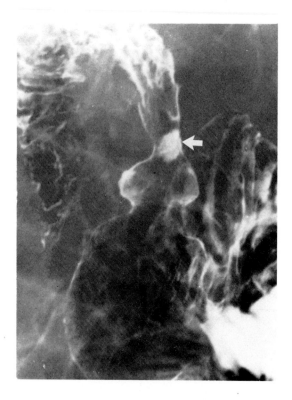

Figure 7.8 Duodenal ulceration associated with some deformity of the cap

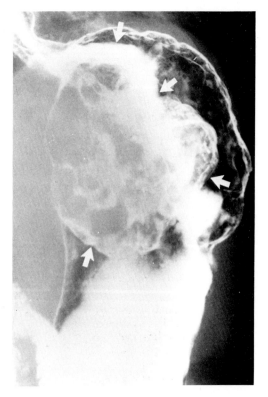

Figure 7.9 Gastric carcinoma. Large irregular polypoid filling defect in the fundus and body of the stomach

Table 7.4 Indications for examination of the small intestine

Symptoms	Causes	Radiological features
Abdominal pain, loss of weight, diarrhoea	Crohn's disease	Inflammatory bowel disease producing a variety of appearances Strictures 'Rose-thorn' or deep ulceration Cobblestone mucosa (*Figure 7.10*)
		Terminal ileum most often affected, but involvement of any part of the alimentary tract can occur
Colicky abdominal pain, vomiting	Small bowel obstruction, e.g. adhesions	Will localize site of obstruction; occasionally relieves it
Malabsorption e.g. fat, folic acid, vitamin B_{12}, calcium	Gluten induced enteropathy	Appearances are non-specific. Dilatation of loops of small bowel, normal or coarse mucosal folds. Dilution of barium
	Conditions producing stasis of intestinal contents, e.g. diverticulosis (*Figure 7.11*), blind loops, strictures	

Note In a case of suspected coeliac disease a jejunal biopsy must always be carried out to establish the diagnosis.

Indications for contrast examination of the colon

Double contrast examination of the colon is now routinely performed using barium and air and is essential if small polyps are to be diagnosed.

Table 7.5 Indications for contrast examination of the colon

Symptoms	Causes	Radiological features
Change in bowel habit. Blood loss, may be occult. Unexplained anaemia. Abdominal pain	Carcinoma of the colon	Irregular stricture often with 'shouldering' of margins. Destruction of mucosa. Malignant polyps – filling defects within colon (*Figure 7.12*)

Note Caecal carcinoma may be symptomless apart from anaemia.

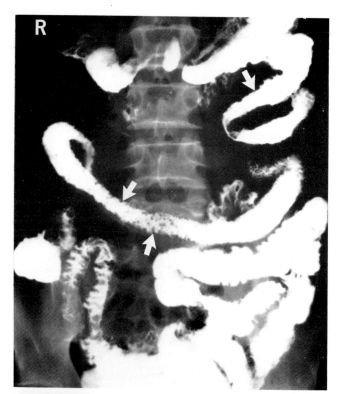

Figure 7.10 Extensive small bowel involvement due to Crohn's disease seen on a barium follow through examination. The abnormalities include deep ulceration and 'cobblestoning' of the mucosa

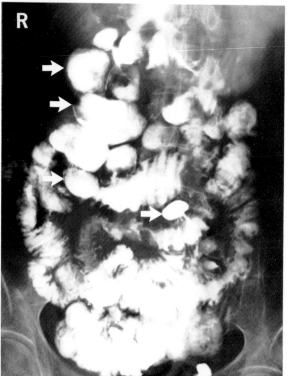

Figure 7.11 Multiple small bowel diverticula

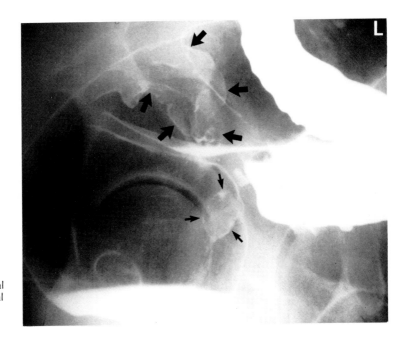

Figure 7.12 Large irregular malignant polyp seen on the posterior rectal wall in a patient presenting with rectal bleeding. The smaller polyp seen anteriorly was benign histologically

Table 7.5 Indications for contrast examination of the colon (continued)

Symptoms	Causes	Radiological features
Abdominal pain, usually left sided. Occasionally diarrhoea and blood loss	Diverticular disease (frequently present in a patient without symptoms)	Multiple diverticula, particularly in pelvic colon. May perforate leading to a surrounding abscess or develop a vesicocolic fistula
Diarrhoea with blood loss. Constitutional disturbance	Ulcerative colitis	Early stage – diffuse fine ulceration, most marked distally. Long standing cases – loss of haustral markings, narrowing and shortening of colon (*Figures 7.13* and *7.14*)
	Ischaemic colitis	Thumb-printing of colonic outline due to oedema and haemorrhage into the mucosa
	Crohn's disease	Areas of narrowing frequently segmental in distribution. Characteristic deep ulceration. Fistulae may be present into small bowel or bladder. Perianal disease is frequent and investigation of the small bowel should also be carried out

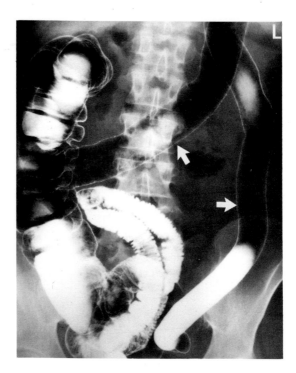

Figure 7.13 Barium enema
examination – appearances typical of
ulcerative colitis. Fine mucosal
ulceration and loss of normal haustral
pattern seen especially well in the
descending and transverse colon

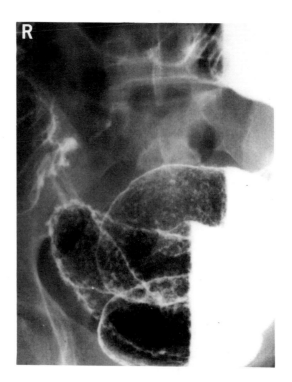

Figure 7.14 Extensive ulceration
involving the rectum and lower
sigmoid colon in a patient with
ulcerative colitis

Table 7.5 Indications for contrast examination of the colon (continued)

Symptoms	Causes	Radiological features
Blood and mucus per rectum Diarrhoea	Polyps Adenomatous polyps	Small polyps usually benign. The larger the polyps the higher the risk of malignancy. Polyps over 2 cm have a high risk of malignancy
	Familial polyposis	Multiple small polyps throughout colon. May be asymptomatic until malignancy supervenes
Watery diarrhoea Hypokalaemia	Villous adenomas	Large pedunculated lesions, distal colon. Frequently become malignant

Note
1. Increased incidence of carcinoma in patients with ulcerative colitis of more than 10 years standing and in severe cases unresponsive to treatment.
2. Familial polyposis – virtually all cases become malignant and careful follow-up of relatives who may develop the condition is essential.
3. Use of colonoscopy allows removal of polyps endoscopically without the need for surgery. Valuable means of following-up and treatment of patients who may develop further polyps.

The biliary tract

Radiological examination is of great value in the investigation of many diseases involving the liver and biliary tract. The particular method used depends on the clinical state of the patient.

Table 7.6 Examination of the biliary tract

Clinical symptoms/signs	Investigation	Radiological features
Attacks of biliary colic or cholecystitis without jaundice	Oral cholecystogram	Most stones are transradiant and show as filling defects within the opacified gall bladder
		Non-opacification of the gall bladder in the presence of normal liver function is virtually diagnostic of gall bladder disease
	Ultrasound	May be performed instead of oral cholecystogram. Valuable to confirm the radiological findings in doubtful cases or if the gall bladder is non-functioning (*Figure 7.15*)
	Intravenous cholangiography	To demonstrate bile ducts if the gall bladder has been removed

Note Neither oral cholecystography nor intravenous cholangiography should be requested in a jaundiced patient as the biliary tract will not be opacified.

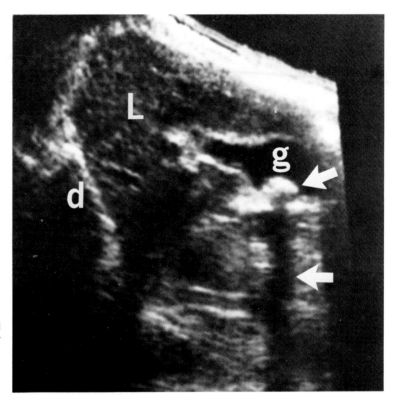

Figure 7.15 Longitudinal ultrasound scan through the right lobe of the liver (L) showing the gall bladder (g). This contains a calculus which reflects the ultrasound beam producing acoustic shadowing beyond

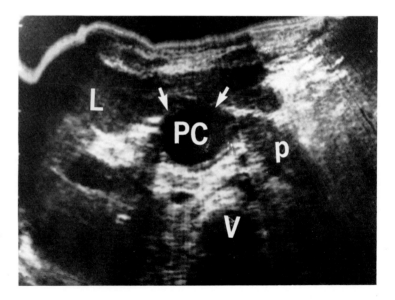

Figure 7.16 Transverse ultrasound scan through the upper abdomen in a patient who has had an attack of acute pancreatitis. The body of the pancreas is seen (p) and a pseudocyst (PC) is present in the head (L = liver; V = vertebral body)

Table 7.6 Examination of the biliary tract (continued)

Clinical symptoms/signs	Investigation	Radiological features
Jaundice	Ultrasound	Demonstrates the gall bladder and the presence or absence of dilatation of the intrahepatic ducts, i.e. can differentiate hepatocellular from obstructive jaundice in majority of cases
	Percutaneous transhepatic cholangiography	Fine needle inserted into the liver and contrast medium injected into the ducts. Valuable investigation to localize the site and nature of the obstruction
	Endoscopic retrograde cholangio-pancreatography (ERCP)	Endoscopic cannulation of the ampulla of Vater and retrograde injection of contrast medium into common bile duct and/or pancreatic duct

Note
1. The hepatorenal syndrome is an absolute contraindication to oral cholecystography and cholangiography.
2. An interval of 4–7 days should elapse between an oral cholecystogram and intravenous cholangiography due to increased toxicity from the combination of the two media.

The pancreas

The demonstration of disease of the pancreas may be difficult radiologically unless there is calcification present, but useful information can be obtained by using other techniques including ultrasound (*Figure 7.16*), computed tomography (*Figure 7.17*), ERCP and selective arteriography.

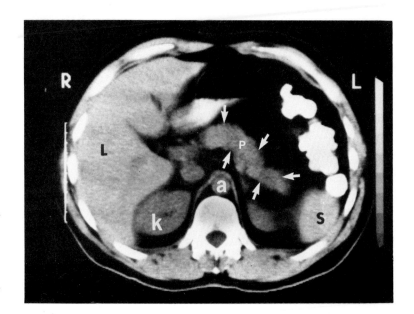

Figure 7.17 CT scan through the upper abdomen demonstrating a normal pancreas, P. The liver, L, spleen S, right kidney, k and aorta, a, are also seen

Chapter 8   The genitourinary system

Examination of the genitourinary system

Although some information may be obtained about the genitourinary system from plain abdominal radiographs, iodine-containing water soluble contrast media are administered intravenously in order to demonstrate the pelvicalyceal systems, the ureters and the bladder satisfactorily. Excretion urography and other contrast examinations of the genitourinary tract, such as micturating cystography, ascending urethrography, hysterosalpingography are directly controlled or supervised by a radiologist in order to obtain the maximum amount of information from each examination.

Procedures involving the use of contrast media should not be carried out lightly on any patient: there must always be a strong clinical indication before these are requested, as all the iodine containing contrast media may cause hypersensitivity reactions varying from mild skin rashes to anaphylaxis and death. It is not generally possible to predict which patients will react in this way, but there is occasionally a history of atopic disease, such as asthma or hay fever, or a known previous hypersensitivity reaction to contrast medium.

Note If excretion urography is necessary in such a patient, prior corticosteroid cover must be given.

Contrast examinations employed in the genitourinary tract

Excretion urography

This is generally carried out when disease of the kidneys, ureters or bladder is suspected, or if there is thought to be involvement of the urinary system by adjacent abdominal disease.

The patient is dehydrated for approximately 12 hours prior to the examination and laxatives given to clear overlying colon. In all cases a 'control' plain abdominal radiograph is obtained initially, otherwise opaque calculi may be obscured by the contrast medium in the collecting systems. A series of radiographs are then taken. Shortly after injection the nephrogram phase is seen; the renal parenchyma is well demonstrated at this stage due to the presence of contrast medium in the tubules. Slightly later films will show filling of the calyces and renal pelvis and, generally, the contrast

Note
1. In young children, patients with renal failure, acute renal colic or myelomatosis, dehydration is omitted.
2. It is acceptable to have a slight difference in renal size between the two sides if the outlines are smooth; up to 2 cm may be normal in adults.
3. Tomography is frequently useful if the renal outlines are obscured by overlying bowel gas.

119

medium will be seen in the ureters and bladder about 15 minutes after injection.

If an obstructive uropathy is suspected, delayed films of up to 24 hours or longer are often necessary to delineate the site of obstruction.

Retrograde pyelography

Although now rarely required, this can be carried out in patients with obstructive uropathy if other methods are unavailable.

Antegrade pyelography

This procedure is performed by percutaneous puncture of the renal pelvis and is carried out in patients with hydronephrosis who have a distal obstruction, which may be due to a calculus or possibly a benign or malignant stricture. Following this examination catheters may be left in situ to allow drainage of urine until the obstruction can be surgically relieved, i.e. a percutaneous nephrostomy.

Micturating cystourethrography

This is carried out to look for ureteric reflux in children with urinary tract infection, or urethral valves in young male children with hydronephrosis which may be associated with renal failure. Bladder function may also be assessed, especially if the procedure is combined with pressure studies. This examination, however, entails a high radiation dose to the gonads as well as the risk of introducing infection during catheterization.

An alternative method of detecting vesicoureteric reflux involves a radiopharmaceutical injected intravenously. This is excreted by the kidneys, filling the bladder. Ureteric reflux can be detected by a gamma camera during micturition.

Ascending urethrography

Generally carried out to assess urethral strictures in males and in cases of pelvic trauma where damage to the urethra is suspected.

Hysterosalpingography

Mainly performed for the investigation of infertility to assess tubal patency or detect uterine malformations.

Table 8.1 Some common anatomical variants seen in the genitourinary tract

Duplex kidney
Horseshoe kidney (*Figure 8.1*)
Crossed renal ectopia
Pelvic kidney
Ureterocoele (*Figure 8.2*)
Urethral valves
Bicornuate uterus (*Figure 8.3*)

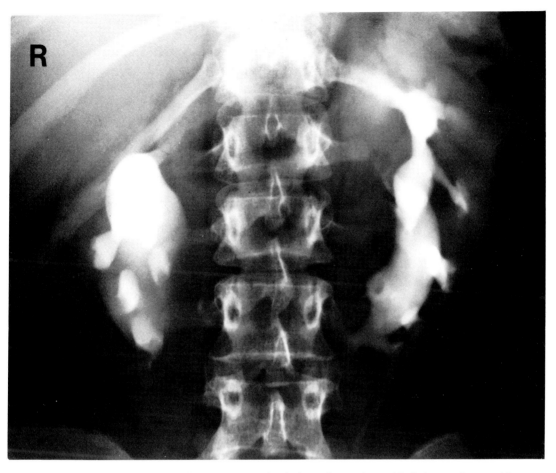

Figure 8.1   Horseshoe kidney. Abnormal axis of the kidneys with some of the calyces pointing medially. The soft tissue bridge between the two lower poles may cause ureteric compression resulting in hydronephrosis

Figure 8.2 (top right)   Ureterocoele. Post micturition radiograph showing the dilated lower end of the ureter – 'cobra head' appearance. A full bladder may conceal this and the patient may be seen to have only a dilated ureter down to the vesicoureteric junction

Figure 8.3 (bottom right)   Hysterosalpingogram showing a bicornuate uterus with two separate cervical canals and uterine bodies. The fallopian tubes are patent – free peritoneal spill of contrast on both sides

121

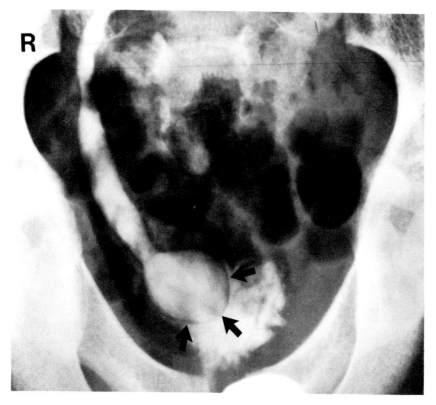

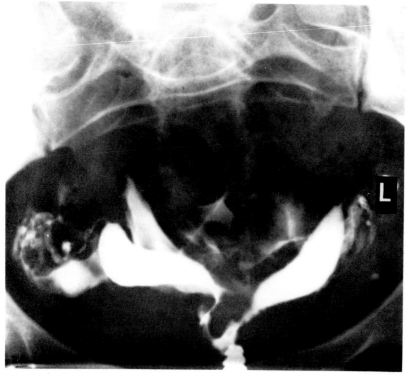

Table 8.2 Common radiological problems related to the urinary tract

	Clinical features	Radiological features
Renal colic		An opaque calculus may be seen on the control radiograph. Signs of obstruction include delay in appearance of the nephrogram on the affected side, dilatation of the collecting system and ureter down to the point of obstruction. Occasionally extravasation of contrast medium is seen around the affected renal pelvis.
		Note Urography should be carried out during an attack of colic if possible. This gives the best chance of detecting ureteric obstruction as these changes may resolve within hours of passing a calculus. After passage of a small ureteric calculus the only abnormal sign may be oedema of the affected ureteric orifice and distension of the lower ureter.
Renal failure		Ultrasound is a most useful initial investigation: to assess renal size and shape to exclude post renal obstruction Excretion urography using high doses of contrast media and tomographic cuts may be performed
Renal mass	This is a relatively common diagnostic problem. The patient may present with haematuria, a palpable abdominal mass – generally in children or thin adults only – or a mass may be discovered incidentally in a patient undergoing an excretion urogram for some unrelated condition, e.g. prostatism.	Excretion urography Enlarged kidney or localized bulge of its outline. Compressed, stretched or missing calyces (*Figure 8.4*). Renal displacement, or ureteric deviation if the mass is large and mainly extrarenal (*Figure 8.5*). Occasionally, absent nephrogram in the affected portion of the kidney (For further radiological investigation *see Figure 8.6*)
Renal tract injury Kidney and ureter	Haematuria and loin pain	Frequently evidence of skeletal injury, e.g. fracture of transverse processes or lower ribs
		Non-function may indicate damage to renal artery. Defect in renal outline and calyceal abnormalities seen if kidney is transected. Renal contusion – may only see blood clot which appears as filling defect in the renal pelvis
		Extravasation of contrast medium if the ureter is avulsed or if there is a tear in the renal cortex and capsule
		Note The main indication for excretion urography in trauma is to assess the presence and function of the contralateral kidney, particularly if surgery on the injured kidney is contemplated.

123

Bladder/Urethra	Generally associated pelvic fractures. Anuria or haematuria	Bladder may be displaced or compressed by a pelvic haematoma. If urethral damage is suspected, ascending urethrography using water soluble contrast medium is carried out
Hypertension	Renal disorders Chronic pyelonephritis	Shrunken scarred kidneys
	Chronic glomerulonephritis	Small smooth kidneys
	Polycystic kidneys (Figures 8.5, 8.8), may be associated with cysts in the liver and pancreas or congenital intracranial berry aneurysms	Both kidneys are large, frequently palpable clinically. At excretion urography numerous cysts seen displacing and stretching the calyces and infundibula. Ultrasound is of great value in the detection of renal cysts and associated cysts in other organs
	Renal artery stenosis	At excretion urography the affected kidney tends to be smaller but its outline is smooth. There is a delay in the appearance of the nephrogram on the affected side – seen best on early films. Ureteric notching may be present due to collateral circulation. The degree of stenosis may be determined by angiography and, in some patients, relief of the hypertension may follow dilatation of the stenosed artery, i.e. transluminal angioplasty. Isotope studies are also of value in this condition, showing a decrease of perfusion on the affected side
	Endocrine disorders Phaeochromocytoma (Figures 8.9a and b)	A soft tissue mass may be seen above the kidney. CT scanning is now the method of choice in the investigation of adrenal tumours
	Hyperaldosteronism (Conn's Syndrome) Cushing's Syndrome	In adrenal tumours venous sampling under radiological control will detect elevated hormone levels

Note In a large majority of patients presenting with hypertension, especially the middle aged and elderly, no cause will be found. Radiological studies should be reserved for the young patient or those in whom clinical or biochemical evidence suggests a remedial cause.

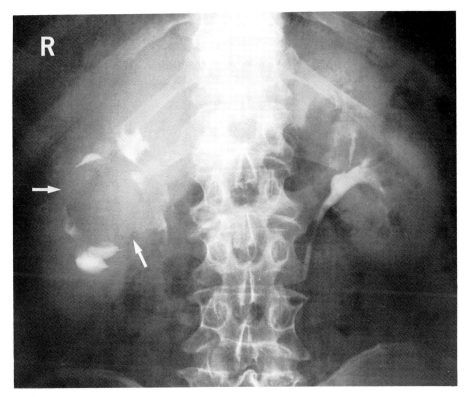

Figure 8.4 Intravenous pyelogram showing a space occupying lesion in the middle of the right kidney – the pelvicalyceal system is compressed and displaced by the mass

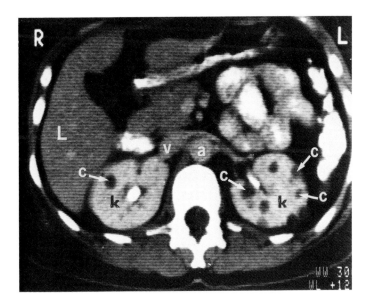

Figure 8.5 CT scan showing cysts (c) bilaterally in the kidneys (k). The left renal vein passes anterior to the aorta (a) and enters the inferior vena cava (v). The liver, L, is also demonstrated

Figure 8.6 Investigation of a renal mass detected during excretion urography

Ultrasound scan

Cystic

Solid

Solitary

↓

Simple cyst has characteristic appearances. Transonic area with clearly defined walls

↓

± Cyst puncture

to obtain fluid for cytology if in doubt

Multiple, bilateral, i.e. polycystic kidneys. The liver and pancreas are examined for associated cysts.

Most commonly suggests a renal carcinoma (*Figure 8.7*), but inflammatory masses may also appear solid.

↓

Angiography   or   Computed tomography

± Therapeutic embolization

Renal carcinoma is usually very vascular at angiography

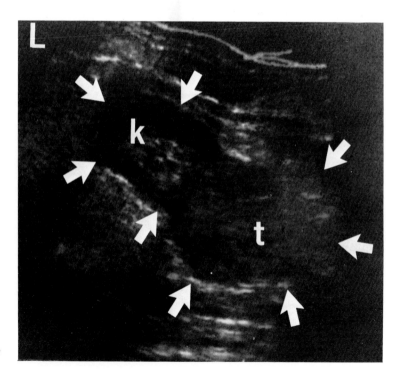

Figure 8.7   Ultrasound scan through the left kidney (K) showing a mass containing echoes related to the lower pole. This is characteristic of a renal tumour (t). The normal upper pole of the kidney and calyceal pattern can be seen

126

Polycythaemia

A condition in which there is overproduction of red blood cells. It may be primary, i.e. polycythaemia rubra vera, where the cause is unknown, or secondary. Several disorders affecting the kidney may give rise to polycythaemia, e.g. carcinoma, polycystic kidneys and hydronephrosis. Non-renal causes include hepatomas, cerebellar haemangioblastomas and uterine fibroids, as well as chronic pulmonary disease.

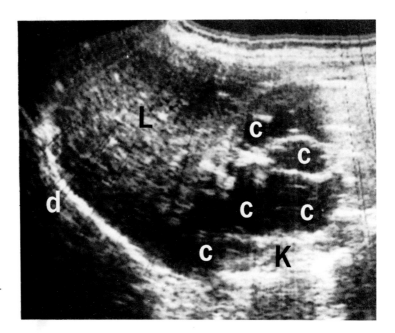

Figure 8.8 Ultrasound scan of the right kidney (K) showing numerous cysts (c) present in a patient with polycystic kidneys – no cysts seen within the liver (L)

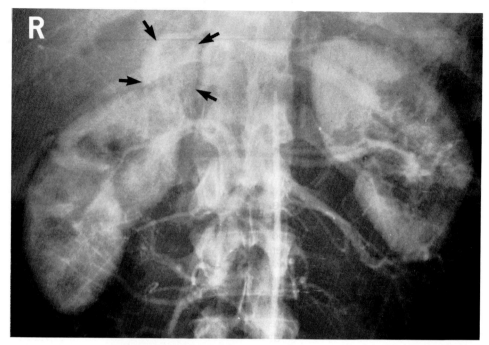

Figure 8.9a Phaeochromocytoma – right adrenal gland. Angiogram shows the vascular adrenal tumour above the right kidney

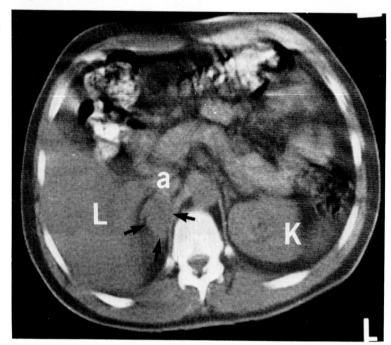

Figure 8.9b CT scan of the same patient also demonstrates the tumour in the right adrenal gland (a)

Chapter 9

Blood vessels and lymphatics

The vascular system

Blood vessels are not shown unless their walls are calcified. Therefore, arteriography must be performed to estimate the extent of vascular disease, atheromatous plaques or occlusions. An artery, generally the femoral, is punctured under local anaesthetic, and a catheter is introduced over a guidewire into the vessel under fluoroscopic control. Water soluble contrast medium is then injected under pressure and films are obtained of the region to be studied. It is possible to inject embolic materials such as Gelfoam through the catheter to control bleeding or cut down the blood supply to a very vascular tumour prior to surgery.

Peripheral vascular disease

Arteriography shows the extent and exact site of vessel involvement in cases of peripheral vascular disease affecting the lower limb (*Figure 9.1*). Before vascular reconstruction or a bypass procedure is attempted, the surgeon needs to know the collateral circulation present, if and where the artery is reconstituted and whether there is a good distal blood flow below the popliteal artery (*Figure 9.2*).

A history of sudden onset of pain in a limb, followed by pallor, decreased skin temperature and absent peripheral pulses clinically indicate an embolic episode; arteriography will localize the site of the embolus accurately.

If a localized area of stenosis is found at arteriography it is possible to dilate the vessel by means of a balloon catheter, thus avoiding an operation in a patient who may be a poor surgical risk. This procedure is known as transluminal angioplasty.

Abdominal aortic aneurysms

On a plain abdominal radiograph, especially the lateral view, calcification may be seen in the wall of the aneurysm which gives some idea as to the external diameter, but not the size of the inner lumen or amount of thrombus present.

Abdominal aortic aneurysms can be fully investigated by computed tomography and ultrasound (*Figure 9.3a and b*) and, where possible, these are the methods of choice.

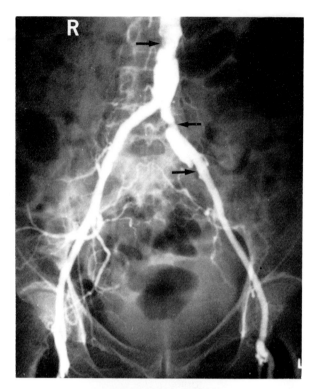

Figure 9.1 Angiogram showing extensive atheroma involving lower aorta and iliac vessels. Plaques and stenoses are present; both internal iliac arteries are occluded

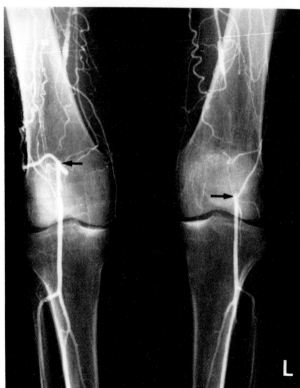

Figure 9.2 Distally, there are blocks in the femoral arteries but collateral channels have opened up and the popliteal arteries on both sides are reconstituted above the knee with a good distal 'run-off'

Note To confirm or exclude the presence of a pulmonary embolism a ventilation and perfusion isotope lung scan should be carried out and not venography.

Deep vein thrombosis

In a clinically difficult case, where a deep vein thrombosis or pulmonary embolism is suspected but clinical evidence of the source of embolism is absent, lower limb venography may be useful in determining the site and extent of the thrombus. This is carried out by injection of water soluble contrast medium into a vein on the dorsum of the foot.

The lymphatic system

The lymph vessels and nodes can be outlined by an oily, radio-opaque medium which is injected slowly into a small lymphatic vessel on the dorsum of the foot. At the end of injection films are taken which demonstrate the opacified lymph vessels of the limbs, pelvis, abdomen and filling of the thoracic duct. A further series of radiographs is obtained about twenty-four hours later which show filling of inguinal, pelvic and para-aortic lymph nodes.

Contraindications to lymphangiography include patients with impaired respiratory function and those who have had recent radiotherapy or an inguinal lymph node biopsy.

The main indications for lymphangiography are staging of reticuloses to allow for optimum treatment planning and, occasionally, detection of metastases, e.g. in bladder carcinoma. Computed tomography, however, now offers an excellent and less invasive method by which lymph node enlargement may be assessed (*Figure 9.4*).

(a)

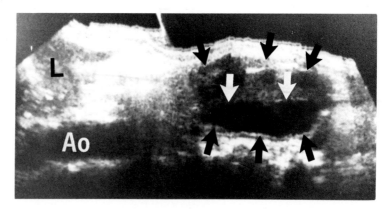

(b)

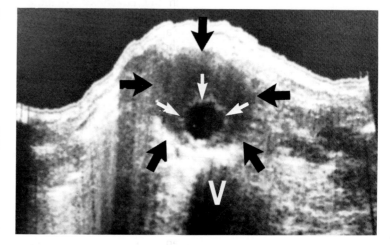

Figure 9.3a and b   Ultrasound scan of the abdominal aorta (Ao). Longitudinal and transverse sections showing the patent central lumen, approximately 2.5 cm in diameter (white arrows), with thrombus formation peripherally. The actual size of the aneurysm is shown by the black arrows and measures approximately 6 cm

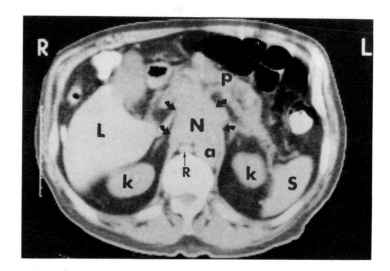

Figure 9.4   CT scan – lymphoma. A large mass of nodes (N) surrounds the aorta (a) and displaces vessels and the pancreas (p) anteriorly. An enlarged retrocrural node (R) is also seen. L represents liver, S spleen and k kidneys

Chapter 10 The nervous system

With the advent of computed tomography, many of the more invasive neuroradiological procedures, such as air encephalography and cerebral angiography, are much less frequently carried out.

The place of skull radiography has already been discussed (*see* Chapter 4).

Intracranial space occupying lesions (*Figure 10.1*)

These may be suspected clinically in a patient who develops focal neurological signs or other evidence of raised intracranial pressure.

The initial investigation of choice which should be carried out in these patients is a CT scan. Apart from being less invasive, sufficient information is frequently obtained to allow both the diagnosis to be made and the appropriate treatment to be planned. No special patient preparation is needed prior to a CT head scan, which is often performed as an outpatient procedure. The head must, however, be immobilized during the scan to avoid motion artefacts; patient cooperation is, therefore, necessary. Water soluble contrast medium may be administered intravenously if a lesion is seen on the initial 'cuts' obtained. If the lesion is vascular it tends to 'enhance', often in a characteristic fashion, e.g. a glioma will show irregular enhancement, meningiomas generally a very marked enhancement, and brain abscesses tend to enhance around the margins of the abscess. In addition, the amount of associated cerebral oedema present can be determined on the CT scan, as can the degree of midline shift and ventricular compression.

Following the CT scan, arteriography may be necessary to demonstrate the vascular supply of the tumour pre-operatively.

Subarachnoid haemorrhage

The majority of cases are caused by rupture of an intracranial aneurysm. These are frequently small and located around the circle of Willis. Bleeding may also occur from an arterio-venous malformation.

133

Clinically these patients present with headache, neck stiffness and altered level of consciousness or neurological signs, e.g. a third nerve palsy due to pressure from a posterior communicating aneurysm. A lumbar puncture will reveal blood stained cerebro-spinal fluid following a subarachnoid haemorrhage.

Although a CT scan in the early stages after a bleed will frequently show intracerebral blood clot and blood in the ventricles, angiography is necessary to determine the exact site of the aneurysm and to see whether multiple aneurysms are present. If an arterio-venous malformation is present its vascular supply and the draining vessels can be accurately shown by angiography.

Trauma

Acute (Figure 10.2)

Following head injuries, CT scanning will reveal the extent of intracranial damage, e.g. the site and size of a haematoma and the degree of midline shift it may be causing.

Chronic

Subdural haematomas in the elderly may be seen some time after the initial injury, which may have been relatively trivial and forgotten. These patients clinically deteriorate slowly, frequently becoming confused or developing localized neurological signs.

CT has generally replaced angiography in making the diagnosis of this condition. In long standing cases low density subdural collections are seen. These have a characteristic shape and compress the underlying brain.

Myelography

Intervertebral disc protrusion or tumours of the spinal cord may not be revealed on plain radiographs of the spine. Myelography is therefore necessary to outline the subarachnoid space and identify nerve roots which may be compressed by a prolapsed disc, giving rise to symptoms (*Figure 10.3*).

Tumours within the spinal canal also cause symptoms because of cord compression and in these cases myelography is necessary to outline the spinal cord to enable the exact level of the lesion to be determined.

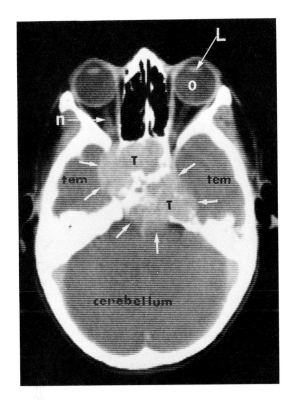

Figure 10.1 CT scan of a pituitary tumour. There is a large irregular soft tissue mass (T) arising from the pituitary fossa and invading both brain and bone. O = orbit, L = lens, n = optic nerve, tem = temporal lobe

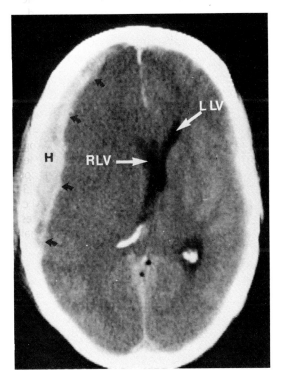

Figure 10.2 CT scan of a subdural haematoma (H). This shows an area of high density with a fairly straight medial margin lying in the frontoparietal region. The right lateral ventricle (RLV) is compressed and both ventricles are shifted over to the left. The left lateral ventricle (LLV) is seen

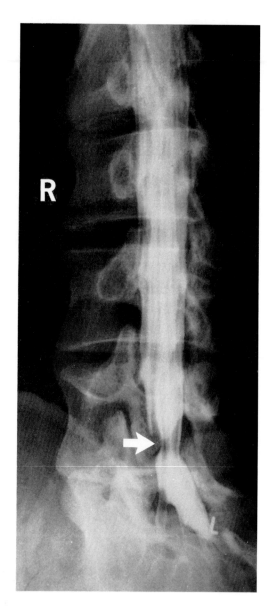

Figure 10.3 Water soluble radiculogram – protrusion of a disc at L.5/S.1 causing nerve root entrapment

Index